MILADY'S STANDARD COSMETOLOGY
THEORY WORKBOOK

MILADY'S STANDARD COSMETOLOGY
THEORY WORKBOOK

TO BE USED WITH

MILADY'S STANDARD COSMETOLOGY

COMPILED BY LISHA BARNES

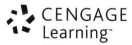
CENGAGE
Learning™

Australia • Brazil • Japan • Korea • Mexico • Singapore • Spain • United Kingdom • United States

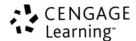

Milady's Standard Cosmetology: Theory Workbook

Compiled by Lisha Barne

For product information and technology assistance, contact us at **Cengage Learning Customer & Sales Support, 1-800-354-9706**

For permission to use material from this text or product, submit all requests online at **cengage.com/permissions** Further permissions questions can be emailed to **permissionrequest@cengage.com**

ISBN-13: 978-1-4180-4941-6

ISBN-10: 1-4180-4941-7

Milady
Executive Woods
5 Maxwell Drive
Clifton Park, NY 12065
USA

Cengage Learning is a leading provider of customized learning solutions with office locations around the globe, including Singapore, the United Kingdom, Australia, Mexico, Brazil, and Japan. Locate your local office at: **international.cengage.com/region**

Cengage Learning products are represented in Canada by Nelson Education, Ltd.

Visit our corporate website at **cengage.com**

Notice to the Reader

Publisher does not warrant or guarantee any of the products described herein or perform any independent analysis in connection with any of the product information contained herein. Publisher does not assume, and expressly disclaims, any obligation to obtain and include information other than that provided to it by the manufacturer. The reader is expressly warned to consider and adopt all safety precautions that might be indicated by the activities described herein and to avoid all potential hazards. By following the instructions contained herein, the reader willingly assumes all risks in connection with such instructions. The publisher makes no representations or warranties of any kind, including but not limited to, the warranties of fitness for particular purpose or merchantability, nor are any such representations implied with respect to the material set forth herein, and the publisher takes no responsibility with respect to such material. The publisher shall not be liable for any special, consequential, or exemplary damages resulting, in whole or part, from the readers' use of, or reliance upon, this material.

Printed in the United States of America
3 4 5 6 7 11 10 09 08

CONTENTS

HOW TO USE THIS WORKBOOK

Milady's Standard Cosmetology Theory Workbook has been written to meet the needs, interests, and abilities of students receiving training in cosmetology.

This workbook should be used together with *Milady's Standard Cosmetology* and *Milady's Standard Cosmetology Practical Workbook.* This book directly follows the theoretical information found in the student textbook. Pages to be read and studied are listed at the beginning of each chapter. The practical information can be found in *Milady's Standard Cosmetology Practical Workbook.*

Students are to answer each item in this workbook with a pencil after consulting their textbook for correct information. Items can be corrected and/or rated during class or individual discussions, or on an independent study basis.

Various tests are included to emphasize essential facts found in the textbook and to measure the student's progress.

HISTORY & CAREER OPPORTUNITIES

Date: _____

Rating: _____

Text Pages: 1-11

POINT TO PONDER:

"Remember, determination, and enthusiasm triumph over talent and laziness every time."—**Life's Little Instruction Calendar**

EARLY HISTORY

1. The term used to encompass a broad range of specialty areas, including hairstyling, nail technology, and esthetics is _____.

2. Define cosmetology: _____

   _____

3. What Greek word is the term cosmetology derived from? _____ What does this term mean? _____

4. Archeological studies reveal that haircutting and hairstyling were practiced in some form as early as the _____.

5. What ordinary items were used as implements and hair adornment during this time?

   _____

6. What natural products did ancient people use for coloring matter and tattooing? _____

   _____

7. Who was the first civilized culture to cultivate beauty into an extravagant fashion? _____
   _____. For what purposes did they use cosmetics? _____

   _____.

8. When was the first evidence of cosmetics in Egypt recorded? _____

    a) 3,000 BC

    b) 2,000 BC

    c) 1,500 BC

    d) 1,000 BC

9. What did Chinese aristocrats rub onto their nails to turn them crimson or ebony?

    _____

10. In 500 BC, during the Golden Age of _____, hairstyling became a highly developed art.

11. Greek women applied preparations of _____ on their faces, _____ on their eyes, and _____ on their cheeks and lips.

12. How did the Greeks create the brilliant red pigment used? _____
    _____.

13. In Rome, women used hair color to indicate their class in society. Match the correct shade with its corresponding class:

    ___ 1) Noblewomen   a) Black

    ___ 2) Middle-class women   b) Red

    ___ 3) Poor women   c) Blond

14. During the Middle Ages, where did women not wear colored makeup? _____

15. What was discouraged during the Renaissance period? _____
    _____.

16. During the Victorian Age, what did women use to preserve the health and beauty of the skin? _____. What were they made from? _____
    _____.

17. To induce natural color rather than use cosmetics, what is it said that Victorian women did? _____.

18. Explain the symbolic meaning of the barber pole. _____
    _____
    _____
    _____
    _____.

19. _____ invented a heavily wired machine that supplied electrical current to metal rods around which hair strands were wrapped.

20. What method of permanent waving was developed in 1941? _____

21. Since the late 1980's, the salon industry has evolved to include _____ .

22. List the various areas you may specialize in within the professional industry:

_____

_____

_____

_____

_____

_____

23. Explain which of the specialized areas you are most interested in and why:

_____

_____

_____

24. List the ways you make each day in school a positive impact on your future:

_____

_____

_____

_____

25. Your license will unlock countless doors, but what two things will fuel your career?

_____

2 LIFE SKILLS

Date: _____

Rating: _____

Text Pages: 12-24

POINT TO PONDER:

Show up! Woody Allen said, 90% of life is "showing up." Go to class—even when you don't feel like it, when the subject matter seems boring, when you have to bum a ride or take the bus because your car died, when you have a bad hair day or a hangover. Go to class!

1. The salon is a creative workplace where you will exercise your artistic talent, and it is a highly social atmosphere that will require _____ and excellent _____ .

2. Below is a list of different life skills. Put a check mark next to the skills you feel you are well on your way to mastering, and put a circle next to the ones you need to improve.

_____ Being genuinely caring and helpful to others

_____ Successfully adapting to different situations

_____ Sticking to a goal and seeing a job to completion

_____ Being consistent with your work

_____ Developing a deep reservoir of common sense

_____ Making good friends

_____ Feeling good about yourself

_____ Maintaining a cooperative attitude

_____ Defining your own code of ethics and living within your definition

_____ Approaching all your work with a strong sense of responsibility

_____ Mastering techniques that will help you become more organized

_____ Having a sense of humor to bring you through difficult situations

_____ Acquiring patience, one of the greatest virtues

_____ Always striving for excellence

3. What must you first do to be successful? _____

4. List the "rules" that will help take you down the road of success:

_____

_____

_____

_____

_____

_____

_____

_____

THE PSYCHOLOGY OF SUCCESS

5. All the talent in the world will not make you successful. What must talent be fueled by in order to sustain your career? _____

6. List the basic principles that form the foundation of all personal and business success:

_____

_____

_____

_____

_____

_____

_____

_____

_____

7. How is self-esteem related to success? _____

_____

8. What will help you turn the possibilities in your life into realities? _____

9. How can you maintain a positive self-image? _____

10. You should not depend on how other people define success. How do you define success?

_____

_____

11. How can you develop success? _____

_____

12. What is a counterproductive activity in the salon? _____

_____

13. Circle the correct answer: Successful stylists do / do not run themselves ragged; they do / do not eat, sleep, and drink beauty. They do / do not take care of their personal needs by spending time with family and friends, having hobbies, and enjoying recreational activities.

14. List three ways to show respect for others:

_____

_____

_____

15. Unscramble these terms and then match them with their definition below.

    naotiostcrinpra   mfepnictsioer   eagm apln

    _____   To put off until tomorrow what you can do today.

    _____   The compulsion to do things perfectly

    _____   The conscious act of planning your life instead of just letting things happen.

MOTIVATION AND SELF MANAGEMENT

16. What is the difference between motivation and self-management? _____

_____

_____

17. The best motivation for you to learn comes from an _____ to grow.

18. Name four guidelines to follow to enhance your creativity.

    a) _____   c) _____

    b) _____   d) _____

19. What does "change your vocabulary" mean? _____
_____ What are some examples? _____

20. Why is it important to not be self-critical? _____
_____

MANAGING YOUR CAREER

21. What is a mission statement, and how is it useful to your personally? _____
_____
_____

22. Write a personal mission statement:

_____

_____

_____

_____

GOAL SETTING

23. What is the purpose of setting goals? _____

24. Why is it important to map out your goals? _____
_____

25. Describe the difference between short-term goals and long-term goals. _____
_____
_____

26. List five short-term goals and five long-term goals and the actions required to achieve them.

Short-Term Goals   Action

_____   _____

_____   _____

_____   _____

_____   _____

_____   _____

Long-Term Goals	Action
_____	_____
_____	_____
_____	_____
_____	_____
_____	_____

TIME MANAGEMENT

27. Read through the list of time management techniques. Rate each as either a personal strength or an area you need to develop or improve.

Time Management Techniques	Strength	Development Opportunity
Prioritizing tasks		
Designing my own time management system		
Not taking on more than I can handle		
Learning problem solving techniques		
Giving myself free time to regroup		
Taking notes of my thoughts and ideas		
Making schedules for my regular commitments		
Rewarding myself for good work		
Using to-do lists to prioritize tasks and activities		
Making time management a habit		

STUDY SKILLS

28. If you find studying overwhelming what can you do? _____

29. What can you do if you find your mind wanders in class? _____
_____

30. List the habits you can develop to improve your study skills.

_____

_____

_____

_____

_____

_____

_____

_____

ETHICS

31. The moral principles by which we live and work are _____ .

32. List the five ways to show you are ethical.

    1. _____

    2. _____

    3. _____

    4. _____
       _____

    5. _____
       _____

33. Describe how to maintain your integrity: _____
_____

PERSONALITY DEVELOPMENT AND ATTITUDE

34. What are the "ingredients" of a healthy, well-developed attitude? _____
_____
_____

35. What does it mean to be tactful? _____

3 YOUR PROFESSIONAL IMAGE

Date: _____

Rating: _____

Text Pages: 25-32

POINT TO PONDER:

> *"Every day you do one of two things: build health or produce disease in yourself."—Adella Davis*

1. In your own words, explain why image and the way you present yourself will affect your career in the image business:

   _____

   _____

   _____

BEAUTY AND WELLNESS

2. What does being well groomed begin with? _____

3. It is not necessary to do which of the following every day?

   ____ a) Shower or bathe

   ____ b) Be neat and clean

   ____ c) Wear perfume

   ____ d) Use deodorant

4. Most clients will tell you that you smell offensive.

   ____ True

   ____ False

5. _____ is the daily maintenance of cleanliness by practicing good sanitary habits.

6. Working as a stylist behind the chair or doing makeup, nail care, or skin care means that you must be extremely meticulous about your hygiene.

____ True

____ False

7. One of the best ways to ensure that you always smell fresh and clean is to create a _____ to keep in your station or locker. List the items that should be included: _____

_____

8. What should you do if you smoke? _____

_____

LOOKING GOOD

9. An extremely important element of your professional image is

____ a) A cell phone

____ b) Expensive shears

____ c) Well-groomed hair, skin, and nails

____ d) A designer outfit

10. How often should you change your style? _____
_____ Why? _____

11. Why do many salons have a no-fragrance policy for staff members? _____

_____

_____

12. Salon owners and managers view _____ , _____ and _____ as being just as important as technical knowledge and skills.

13. What is one of the most vital aspects of good personal grooming? _____

_____

14. Explain why it is a good idea to invest in an apron or a smock. _____

_____

15. How can you make the best clothing choices that promote your career as a promising stylist? _____

16. What type of shoes are generally recommended? _____

_____

17. Make-up should be used to _____ your best features and _____ your less flattering ones.

YOUR PHYSICAL PRESENTATION

18. _____ is an important part of your physical presentation. Why? _____

_____

_____

19. List the guidelines for achieving and maintaining good standing posture:

_____

_____

_____

_____

_____

20. Define ergonomics: _____

_____

_____

21. Give an example of fitting the job to the person in the salon. _____

_____

_____

22. Cosmetologists are susceptible to problems of the hands, wrists, shoulders, neck, back, feet, and legs, which if not attended to can become career threatening.

____ True

____ False

23. After your next practical service, analyze yourself to see if you do any of the following:

____ Grip or squeeze implements too tightly

____ Bend the wrist up or down constantly when using your tools

____ Hold your arms away from your body as you work

____ Hold your elbows more than a 60-degree angle away from your body for extended periods of time

____ Bend forward and/or twist your body to get closer to your client

24. What measures can you take to avoid these problems?

_____

_____

_____

_____

_____

25. How can you counter the problem of working in an environment that has physical discomfort? _____

_____

26. You should always put your health first and the task at hand second.

___ True

___ False

4 COMMUNICATING FOR SUCCESS

Date: _____

Rating: _____

Text Pages: 33-52

POINT TO PONDER:

> *"Wisdom is knowing when to speak your mind and when to mind your speech."—Evangel*

1. List three things that effective communication skills will help:

   a) _____

   b) _____

   c) _____

HUMAN RELATIONS

2. The key to operating effectively in many professions is to _____ .
   Why is it especially true for cosmetologists? _____

3. The best way to understand others is to begin with a firm understanding of

   ____ a) The salon

   ____ b) State law

   ____ c) Yourself

   ____ d) Your coworkers

4. What are good relationships built on? _____

5. List the emotions we feel when we feel secure. _____ List the
   emotions we feel when we feel insecure. _____

   _____

6. How can you help people around you feel secure? _____

   _____

7. List the ways to handle the ups and downs of human relations and explain what each one means to you:

Explanation

_____

_____

_____

_____

_____

_____

_____

_____

_____

_____

_____

_____

_____

_____

_____

8. The deciding factor in whether or not a relationship is going to be rewarding or demoralizing is how much the other party is willing to give.

____ True

____ False

9. List the guidelines to keep in mind for effective human relations:

a) _____

b) _____

c) _____

d) _____

e) _____

f) _____

g) _____

h) _____

i) _____

j) _____

k) _____

l) _____

COMMUNICATION BASICS

10. Define communication: _____

_____

11. Besides communicating with words, how else do we communicate? _____

_____

12. What is one of the most important communications you will have with a client? _____

_____

13. The first time you meet a client you should be

____ a) Polite, friendly, aloof

____ b) Polite, friendly, inviting

____ c) Friendly, inviting, distant

____ d) Casual, friendly, distant

14. Explain the steps you need to take to earn the client's trust and loyalty:

a) _____

b) _____

c) _____

d) _____

e) _____

15. An intake form that is completed by every new client prior to service may also be called a

_____ or a _____ .

16. In some cosmetology schools, the consultation card may be accompanied by a _____ _____ . What is its purpose? _____

_____

_____

17. What is the purpose of the client consultation? _____

_____

18. The client consultation is the single most important part of any service.

____ True

____ False

19. How often should a client consultation be performed?

____ a) Never

____ b) Every visit

____ c) Every other visit

____ d) Only for chemical services

20. How can you ensure your time is well spent during the client consultation? _____

21. What tools should you prepare for use in the client consultation?

a) _____

b) _____

22. Do all services require the same degree of consultation? _____ Provide an example:

_____

23. The following list is the 10-step consultation. In the space provided, list what you should do during each step.

10 Steps	Action Taken
1. Review	_____
2. Assess	_____
3. Preference	_____
	_____
4. Analyze	_____
	_____
5. Lifestyle	_____

6. Show and tell _____

7. Suggest _____

8. Color _____

9. Upkeep _____

10. Repeat _____

24. At the conclusion of the service, what information should you record on the consultation card? _____

_____

SPECIAL ISSUES IN COMMUNICATION

25. Sometimes you will encounter situations beyond your control. What is the solution?

_____

26. Explain why tardy clients create a problem. _____

_____

27. List ways in which tardy clients can be handled so that you don't lose their business or ruin your day's schedule.

a) _____

b) _____

c) _____

28. When a scheduling mix-up occurs, you should

____ Not admit that you or anyone in the salon made a mistake

____ Argue with the client about who wrote the appointment down wrong

____ Be polite and never argue the point of which one of you is correct

____ Blame the salon receptionist and call the manager

29. Once you master all your hairdressing skills, you will never have an unhappy client.

____ True

____ False

30. Which of the following are appropriate ways of dealing with unhappy clients? (Check all that apply)

    ____ Find out why the client is unhappy

    ____ Do not change what the client dislikes until his or her next visit

    ____ Tactfully explain the reasons why you cannot make changes

    ____ Argue with the client or force your opinion

    ____ Call on a more experienced stylist or salon manager for help

31. It would be unwise to become your client's counselor, career guide, parental sounding board, or motivational coach.

    ____ True

    ____ False

IN-SALON COMMUNICATION

32. Behaving in a _____ is the first step in making this meaningful communication possible.

33. In the salon community, working closely for long hours with your coworkers, it is important to maintain _____ around what you will and will not do or say in the salon.

34. What guidelines should you keep in mind as you interact and communicate with fellow staffers?

    a) _____

    b) _____

    c) _____

    d) _____

    e) _____

    f) _____

    g) _____

35. What things should you strive for when dealing with your manager?

    a) _____

    b) _____

c) _____

d) _____

e) _____

f) _____

36. What kinds of salons conduct frequent and thorough employee evaluations?

   _____

37. It is acceptable for you to ask to see the criteria on which you will be evaluated.

   ____ True

   ____ False

38. Should you rate yourself in the weeks and months ahead of your evaluation? _____
   Why? _____

39. Why do many professionals never take advantage of this crucial communication
   opportunity? _____

40. At the end of the meeting, you should _____

   _____

5 INFECTION CONTROL: PRINCIPLES & PRACTICES

Date: _____

Rating: _____

Text Pages: 54-83

POINT TO PONDER:

"One pound of learning requires ten pounds of common sense to apply it."
—Persian Proverb

1. Explain in your own words why it is important to study infection control. _____
_____
_____
_____

REGULATION
_____

2. In regards to regulating the practice of cosmetology, what is the difference between federal agencies and state agencies? _____
_____
_____

3. Define OSHA. _____

4. OSHA was created as part of the US Department of Labor in order to _____
_____

5. What is the purpose of the Hazard Communication Act? _____
_____

6. What does a Material Safety Data Sheet include? _____
_____
_____
_____

7. What does the Environmental Protection Agency (EPA) license? _____
_____

8. What two types are used in salons?

   a) _____

   b) _____

9. If you do not follow the instructions for mixing contact time and the type of surface the disinfecting product can be used on, you've broken federal law.

   ___ a) True

   ___ b) False

10. Why do state regulatory agencies exist? _____

    _____

11. State agencies rules are enforced through _____ and investigations of consumer complaints.

12. What is the difference between laws and rules? _____

    _____

    _____

PRINCIPLES OF INFECTION

13. List the three types of potentially infectious microorganisms that are important in the practice of cosmetology.

    a) _____

    b) _____

    c) _____

14. Disinfectants used in the salon must be _____ and _____.
    What does that mean? _____

    _____

15. Explain why the cosmetologist is obligated to provide safe services in the salon.

    _____

    _____

16. One-celled microorganisms with both plant and animal characteristics are known as _____. Where can they exist? _____

    _____

17. The vast majority of bacteria which are completely harmless and do not produce disease are _____ organisms.

18. List some of the useful functions of this harmless bacteria.

    a) _____

    b) _____

    c) _____

19. Pathogenic bacteria are harmful because they may cause _____ or infection when they enter the body.

20. Match each term with its correct definition

    ____ 1. microbes/germs   a) Poisonous substances produced by some microorganisms

    ____ 2. microorganism   b) One-celled microorganisms

    ____ 3. parasite   c) Organism of microscopic to submicroscopic size

    ____ 4. bacteria   d) Infection spread from one person to another

    ____ 5. virus   e) An organism that lives on another organism

    ____ 6. infectious   f) Synonyms for any disease-producing bacteria

    ____ 7. toxin   g) Microorganism capable of infecting almost all plants and animals

21. Match each of the following bacteria with its unique shape.

    ____ 1. Cocci   a) Curved lines

    ____ 2. Staphylococci   b) Spiral or corkscrew

    ____ 3. Streptococci   c) Short, rod shaped

    ____ 4. Diplococci   d) Round shape

    ____ 5. Bacilli   e) Grape like clusters

    ____ 6. Spirilla   f) Spherical

22. Pus forming bacteria that causes abscesses, pustules and boils is known as

_____ .

23. Pus forming bacteria that causes infections such as strep throat and blood poisoning is known as _____ .

24. Diplococci is a bacteria that causes diseases such as _____ .

25. How do the following bacteria move about?

    a) Cocci   _____

    b) Bacilla   _____

    c) Spirilla   _____

26. Bacteria move in different ways, motility, which is _____ and _____ or cilia, a whip like motion, which moves the bacteria in liquid.

27. Unscramble these words and use them to complete the sentences below.

briateac   sopotparlm   aticve   cniatvie

_____ generally consist of an outer cell wall containing a liquid called _____. They manufacture their own food from the surrounding environment, give off waste products, and grow and reproduce. The life cycle of bacteria is made up of two distinct phases: the _____ stage, and the _____ or spore-forming stage.

28. During the active stage, bacteria:

____ a) change color

____ b) die

____ c) grow

____ d) dry out

29. The division of bacteria cell is called _____ . The cells that are formed are called

_____

30. What happens to bacteria in favorable conditions? _____ . What happens in unfavorable conditions? _____

31. Why do certain bacteria, such as anthrax and tetanus bacilli, coat themselves with wax outer shells? _____

32. What happens when favorable conditions are restored? _____

_____

33. What occurs when body tissues are invaded by disease-causing or pathogenic bacteria?

_____

34. What is pus? _____

_____

35. Staphylococci are among the most common human bacteria and are normally carried by what percentage of the population?

____ a) ⅛

____ b) ½

____ c) ⅓

____ d) ¼

36. How is a staph infection most frequently transferred? _____

37. Staph infections occur most frequently in people who have _____ immune systems. The symptoms usually appear as skin infections such as: _____ .

38. A _____ is one that is confined to a particular part of the body and is indicated by a lesion containing pus.

39. A disease that spreads from one person to another by contact is said to be contagious or _____.

40. List the more common contagious diseases that will prevent a cosmetologist from servicing a client. _____

41. A _____ is a microorganism capable of infecting almost all plants and animals, including bacteria. They cause:

a) _____

b) _____

c) _____

d) _____

e) _____

f) _____

g) _____

h) _____

i) _____

j) _____

k) _____

l) _____

42. What's the difference between bacteria and viruses? _____

_____

_____

43. _____ can usually be treated with antibiotics while _____ generally are not affected by antibiotics.

44. Vaccination prevents viruses from growing in the body, but are not available for all viruses.

____ True

____ False

45. Disease-causing bacteria or viruses that are carried through the body in the blood or body fluids are called _____ .

List the three types of hepatitis: _____

46. What does HIV stand for? _____

47. What does AIDS stand for? _____ What is AIDS?

_____

48. Is it possible to have HIV for many years and have no symptoms?

____ a) Yes

____ b) No

49. How is the HIV virus transmitted?

a) _____

b) _____

c) _____

50. Name some ways in which the HIV virus is not transmitted. _____

_____

51. _____ are organisms that live in, or on, another _____ organism and draw their _____ from that organism or _____ .

52. _____ which include molds, mildews, and yeasts can produce _____ diseases, such as ringworm.

53. _____ is the most frequently encountered infection resulting from hair services. What does it affect? _____

_____

54. Nail fungus can be spread through _____ implements or when the natural nail is not properly _____ before the enhancement is applied. Nail fungus is usually a _____ condition that is _____ but can spread to other nails or clients if implements are not properly _____ after each service.

55. What should a client do if they are concerned about a fungal infection of the nails?

_____

56. Pathogenic bacteria or viruses or fungi can enter the body through

    a) _____

    b) _____

    c) _____

    d) _____

    e) _____

57. The body prevents and controls infections with

    a) _____

    b) _____

    c) _____

    d) _____

58. Match each of the following terms with its correct definition.

    ____ 1. immunity   a) both inherited and developed through healthy living

    ____ 2. natural immunity   b) ability to overcome disease through inoculation

    ____ 3. acquired immunity   c) the body's ability to destroy and resist infection

6 GENERAL ANATOMY AND PHYSIOLOGY

Date: _____

Rating: _____

Text Pages: 84-118

POINT TO PONDER

"You will never change your life until you change something you do daily. The secret of your success is found in your daily routine."—John C. Maxwell

1. As a cosmetologist, understanding the concept of human anatomy is primarily restricted to

   _____

   _____ .

2. List the reasons a cosmetologists studies anatomy and physiology:

   a) _____

   b) _____

   c) _____

   _____

CELLS _____

3. The basic unit of all living things, from bacteria to plants and animals, including human

   beings are _____ .

4. The cells of all living things are composed of a substance called _____

   a colorless jellylike substance.

5. Match the following terms with the correct definition:

   ____ 1. Anatomy   a) The study of the functions and activities performed by the body structures

   ____ 2. Physiology   b) The dense active protoplasm, found at the center of the cell

   ____ 3. Histology   c) The protoplasm of the cell that surrounds the nucleus

   ____ 4. Nucleus   d) The study of the human body; the science of structure of organisms or of their parts

___ 5. Cytoplasm   e) The balloon to contain the protoplasm, allowing certain substances to pass through

___ 6. Cell membrane   f) The study of the many tiny structures found in living tissue; microscopic anatomy

6. Cells have the ability to reproduce, providing new cells for the growth and replacement of worn or injured one.

___ True

___ False

7. Most cells reproduce by dividing into to two identical cells called _____ . This process of cell reproduction is known as _____ .

8. For cells to grow and reproduce, conditions must be _____ , which include a/an:

a) _____

b) _____

c) _____

9. What will occur if conditions are unfavorable? _____

10. What conditions are considered unfavorable? _____

11. Identify the parts of the cell illustrated:

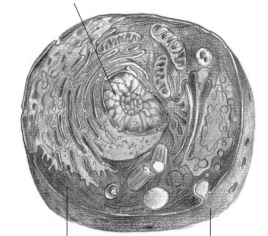

12. _____ is a chemical process that takes place in living organisms, whereby the cells are nourished and carry out their activities.

13. List and define the two phases of metabolism:

    a) _____

    b) _____

    _____

14. During which phase is energy released that has been stored? _____

15. During which phase does the body store water, food, and oxygen? _____

16. Anabolism and catabolism are not carried out simultaneously.

    ___ True

    ___ False

TISSUES

17. A collection of similar cells that perform a particular function are _____.
    Each has a specific function and can be recognized by its _____ appearance.

18. How many types of tissue are there in the body? _____

19. The tissue that is a protective covering on body surfaces is _____.

    a) Liquid

    b) Connective

    c) Epithelial

    d) Muscular

    e) Nerve

20. The tissue that contracts and moves the various parts of the body is _____.

    a) Liquid

    b) Connective

    c) Epithelial

    d) Muscular

    e) Nerve

21. The tissue that serves to support, protect, and bind together other tissues of the body is

   _____.

   a) Liquid

   b) Connective

   c) Epithelial

   d) Muscular

   e) Nerve

22. Tissues such as blood and lymph that carry food, waste products, and hormones through the body are _____.

   a) Liquid

   b) Connective

   c) Epithelial

   d) Muscular

   e) Nerve

23. The tissues that carry messages to and from the brain and control and coordinate all bodily functions are _____.

   a) Liquid

   b) Connective

   c) Epithelial

   d) Muscular

   e) Nerve

24. List examples of connective tissue: _____

   _____

25. List examples of epithelial tissue: _____

   _____

ORGANS

26. Groups of tissues designed to perform a specific function are _____.

27. _____ are groups of bodily organs acting together to perform one or more functions. There are _____ major systems.

28. Define the functions of the following systems:

    a) Circulatory: _____

    b) Digestive: _____

    c) Endocrine: _____

    _____

    d) Excretory: _____

    e) Integumentary: _____

    _____

    f) Muscular: _____

    g) Nervous: _____

    h) Reproductive: _____

    _____

    i) Respiratory: _____

    j) Skeletal: _____

THE SKELETAL SYSTEM

29. _____ is the study of anatomy, structure, and functions of the bones. What prefix used in many medical terms means "bone"? _____

30. The skeletal system is composed of _____ bones that vary in size and shape and are connected by _____ and _____ joints.

31. What other than bone is the hardest tissue in the body? _____

_____

32. List the primary functions of the skeletal system:

    a) _____

    b) _____

    c) _____

    d) _____

e) _____

_____

33. A _____ is the connection between two or more bones of the skeleton. The two types are: _____ .

34. Provide examples of movable joints: _____

35. Provide examples of immovable joints: _____

36. The skull is divided into two parts, the _____ and the _____ which is made up of _____ bones.

37. The cranium is made up of: (_____

    a) 8 bones

    b) 10 bones

    c) 12 bones

    d) 14 bones

38. Match the following bones of the cranium with its correct description:

    ___ 1. Parietal   a) Forms the forehead

    ___ 2. Occipital   b) Hindmost bone of the skull

    ___ 3. Frontal   c) Form the sides of the head in the ear region

    ___ 4. Temporal   d) Form the sides and crown of the cranium

39. Match the following bones of the face with its correct description:

    ___ 1. Nasal   a) Small, thin bones located at the front inner wall

    ___ 2. Lacrimal   b) Lower jawbone, largest and strongest of the face

    ___ 3. Zygomatic   c) Form the bridge of the nose

    ___ 4. Maxillae   d) Bones of the upper jaw

    ___ 5. Mandible   e) Form the prominence of the cheeks

40. Match the following bones of the neck, chest, shoulder, and back with the correct description:

    ___ 1. Hyoid   a) U-shaped bone at the base of the tongue

    ___ 2. Cervical vertebrae b) The chest; elastic, bony cage

    ___ 3. Thorax   c) Shoulder blades

____ 4. Ribs   d) Collarbone

____ 5. Scapula   e) Breastbone

____ 6. Sternum   f) 12 pairs of bones forming the wall of the thorax

____ 7. Clavicle   g) Seven bones of the top part of the vertebral column

41. The smaller bone in the forearm on the same side as the thumb is _____ .

    a) Humerus

    b) Radius

    c) Carpus

    d) Ulna

42. The uppermost and largest bone of the arm is _____ .

    a) Humerus

    b) Radius

    c) Carpus

    d) Ulna

43. The wrist, a flexibile joint composed of a group of eight small, irregular bones

    _____ .

    a) Humerus

    b) Radius

    c) Carpus

    d) Ulna

44. The inner and large bone of the forearm, attached to the wrist and located on the side of the little finger, is the _____ .

    a) Humerus

    b) Radius

    c) Carpus

    d) Ulna

45. The _____ are the bones of the palm of the hand, and the _____ are the bones in the fingers, also called _____ .

46. Match the following terms with the correct definitions:

    ____ 1. Femur   a) Accessory bone; forms the knee cap joint

    ____ 2. Tibia   b) Heavy, long bone; forms the leg above the knee

    ____ 3. Fibula   c) Smaller of two bones, forms the leg below the knee

    ____ 4. Patella   d) Ankle bone of the foot

    ____ 5. Talus   e) Larger of 2 bones, form leg below knee

47. The foot is made up of (_____ bones, subdivided into three categories:

    a) (_____

    b) (_____

    c) (_____

THE MUSCULAR SYSTEM

48. Define the muscular system: _____

_____

49. The study of the structure, function, and disease of the muscles is _____.
The human body has over _____ muscles, which are responsible for approximately
_____ of the body's weight.

50. List the three types of muscular tissue:

    a) _____

    b) _____

    c) _____

51. _____ muscles, also called _____ muscles, are attached to the bones and
are voluntary or controlled by the will.

52. _____ muscles, or _____ muscles, are involuntary and function
automatically, without conscious will.

53. _____ muscles is the involuntary muscle that is the heart.

54. List the two functions of the striated muscles: _____

_____

55. Where are nonstriated muscles found? _____

_____

56. Is the cardiac muscle found anywhere other than the heart?

_____ Yes

_____ No

57. What are the three parts of the muscle? _____ . Define each:

a) _____

b) _____

c) _____

58. To which part of the muscle is pressure applied during massage? _____

59. How is this pressure usually directed? _____

60. List the ways in which muscular tissue can be stimulated:

a) _____

b) _____

c) _____

d) _____

e) _____

f) _____

g) _____

61. Which muscles should the cosmetologists be concerned with? _____

_____

62. The broad muscle that covers the top of the skull is the _____ . It consists of two parts, the _____ and the _____ .

63. The muscle that draws the scalp backward is the _____ .

64. The _____ muscle of the scalp raises the eyebrows, draws the scalp forward, and causes wrinkles across the forehead.

65. What tendon connects the occipitalis and the frontalis? _____

66. Match the muscles of the ear to the correct description:

_____ 1. Auricularis superior   a) Muscle behind the ear that draws the ear backward.

_____ 2. Auricularis anterior   b) Muscle above the ear that draws the ear upward.

_____ 3. Auricularis posterior   c) Muscle in front of the ear that draws the ear forward.

67. The three muscles of the ear have no function.

    ____ True

    ____ False

68. The masseter and the temporalis muscles coordinate the opening and closing of the mouth and are sometimes referred to as the _____ .

69. The broad muscle extending from the chest and shoulder muscles to the side of the chin is the _____ .

70. Which muscle of the neck lowers and rotates the head? _____ .

71. The muscle located beneath the frontalis that draws the eyebrown down is the

    _____ .

    a) Corrugator

    b) Orbicularis oculi

    c) Orbicularis oris

    d) Procerus

72. The muscle that covers the bridge of the nose, lowers the eyebrows and causes wrinkles across the bridge of the nose is the _____ .

    a) Corrugator

    b) Orbicularis oculi

    c) Orbicularis oris

    d) Procerus

73. The muscle that forms the ring of the eye socket, closing the eye is the _____ .

    a) Corrugator

    b) Orbicularis oculi

    c) Orbicularis oris

    d) Procerus

74. Match the following muscles of the mouth with its correct description:

    ____ 1. Buccinator

    ____ 2. Depressor labii inferioris

    a) Muscle that elevates the lower lip and raises and wrinkles the skin of the chin.

    b) Muscles extending from the zygomatic bone to the angle of the mouth, elevate the lip.

____ 3. Levator anguli oris

c) Flat muscle of the cheek between the upper and lower jaw that compresses the cheeks and expels air between the lips.

____ 4. Levator labii superioris

d) A muscle that raises the angle of the mouth and draws it inward.

____ 5. Mentalis

e) Muscle of the mouth that draws the corner of the mouth out and back

____ 6. Orbicularis oris

f) Muscle extending alongside the chin that pulls down the corner of the mouth

____ 7. Risorius

g) A muscle surrounding the lower lip; lowers the lower lip and draws it to one side

____ 8. Triangularis

h) Flat band around the upper and lower lips that compresses, contracts, puckers, and wrinkles the lips

____ 9. Zygomaticus

i) A muscle surrounding the upper lip; elevates the upper lip and dilates the nostrils

75. The broad, flat superficial muscle covering the back of the neck and upper and middle region of the back is the _____.

a) Pectoralis major

b) Serratus anterior

c) Latissimus dorsi

d) Trapezius

76. The muscle that covers the back of the neck and upper middle region of the back and rotates and controls the swinging movements of the arm is the _____.

a) Pectoralis major

b) Serratus anterior

c) Latissimus dorsi

d) Trapezius

77. The muscles of the chest that assist the swinging movements of the arm are the _____.

a) Pectoralis major

b) Serratus anterior

c) Latissimus dorsi

d) Trapezius

78. The muscle of the chest that assists in breathing and in raising the arm is the

_____.

a) Pectoralis major

b) Serratus anterior

c) Latissimus dorsi

d) Trapezius

79. What are the three principal muscles of the shoulders and upper arms? _____

_____

80. Match the following muscle with the correct definition:

____ 1. Biceps
____ 2. Deltoid
____ 3. Triceps
____ 4. Extensors
____ 5. Flexors
____ 6. Pronators
____ 7. Supinator

a) Muscles that straighten the wrist, hand, and fingers to form a straight line

b) Muscle producing the contour of the front and inner side of the upper arm

c) Muscles that turn the hand inward so that the palm faces downward

d) Muscle of the forearm that rotates the radius outward and the palm upward

e) Large triangular muscle covering the shoulder joint

f) Extensor muscles of the wrist; involved in bending the wrist

g) Large muscle that covers the entire back of the upper arm and extends the forearm

81. What is the difference between the abductor and adductor muscles? _____

_____

82. The muscles that bend the foot up and extends the toes is the: _____

a) Peroneus brevis

b) Tibialis anterior

c) Peroneus longus

d) Extensor digitorum longus

83. The muscles that covers the front of the shin and bends the foot upward and inward is the: _____

   a) Peroneus brevis

   b) Tibialis anterior

   c) Peroneus longus

   d) Extensor digitorum longus

84. The muscle that covers the outside of the calf and inverts the foot, turns it outward is the: _____

   a) Peroneus brevis

   b) Tibialis anterior

   c) Peroneus longus

   d) Extensor digitorum longus

85. The muscle that originates at the upper portion of the fibula and bends the foot down is the: _____

   a) Gastrocnemius

   b) Soleus

   c) Peroneus brevis

   d) Peroneus longus

86. The muscle attached to the lower rear surface of the heel and pulls the foot down is the: _____

   a) Gastrocnemius

   b) Soleus

   c) Peroneus brevis

   d) Peroneus logus

87. The muscles of the feet are:

   1. (_____

   2. (_____

   3. (_____

   4. (_____

THE NERVOUS SYSTEM

88. The system that is exceptionally well-organized and is responsible for coordinating all of the many activities that are performed inside and outside the body is the _____ .
_____ .

89. _____ is the scientific study of the structure, function, and pathology of the nervous system.

90. Every square inch of human body is supplied with fine fibers know as _____ .
There are over _____ cells, known as _____ , in the body.

91. Why is it important for a cosmetologist to understand how the nervous system works?
_____
_____

92. What are the principal components of the nervous system? _____
_____

93. List the three main subdivisions of the nervous system.

    a) _____

    b) _____

    c) _____

94. Identify each of the following descriptions as to which subdivision it belongs:

    _____   A system of nerves that connect the outer parts of the body to the central nervous system

    _____   It consists of the brain, spinal cord, spinal nerves, and cranial nerves

    _____   The part of the nervous system that controls the involuntary muscles

    _____   It regulates the action of the smooth muscles, glands, blood vessels, and heart

    _____   It controls consciousness and many mental activities, voluntary functions of the five senses, and voluntary muscle

    _____   It function is to carry impulses, or messages, to and from the central nervous system

95. The _____ is the largest and most complex nerve tissue in the body, is contained in the _____ , and weighs a little less than _____ pounds on average.

96. The portion of the central nervous system that originates in the brain, extends down to the lower extremity of the trunk, and is protected by the spinal column is the _____ _____ . How many pairs of spinal nerves extend from it? _____

97. A _____ is the primary structural unit of the nervous system and is composed of _____ and _____ .

98. Treelike branchings of nerve fibers extending from the nerve cell that receives impulses from other neurons are _____ , and the _____ sends impulses away from the cell body to the other neurons, glands, or muscles.

99. The whitish cords made up of bundles of nerve fibers held together by connective tissue, through which impulses are transmitted are _____ . Where do they have their origin? _____

100. There are _____ types of nerves: _____ , which carry impulses or messages from the sense organs to the brain and _____ , which carry impulses from the brain to the muscles.

101. The sensations of touch, cold, heat, sight, hearing, taste, smell, pain, and pressure are experienced by the _____ nerve.

102. The impulses that produce movement are transmitted by the _____ nerve.

103. Which of the cranial nerves is the largest? _____ List the two additional names for this nerve: _____ . What is the purpose of this nerve: _____
_____

104. List the branches of the fifth cranial nerve that are affected by massage and explain what area is affected:

a) (_____
_____

b) (_____
_____

c) (_____

d) (_____

e) (_____

f) (_____

g) (_____

105. The motor nerve of the face is the _____ cranial nerve.

106. List the most important branches of the facial nerve:

    a) (_____

    b) (_____

    c) (_____

    d) (_____

    e) (_____

    f) (_____

107. The principle nerves supplying the superficial parts of the arm and hand are the _____ _____ , and the _____ .

108. Identify the nerves of the arm and hand illustrated below:

109. The nerve that supplies impulses to the knee, the muscles of the calf, the skin of the leg and the sole, heel and underside of the toes is the _____ .

110. Match the following terms with the correct definition.

    ___ 1. Common peroneal   a) Extends down the leg, supplies impulses to the muscles and skin of the leg.

    ___ 2. Deep peroneal nerve   b) Extends from behind the knee to wind around the head of the fibula to the front of the leg

    ___ 3. Superficial peroneal nerve   c) Extends down to the front of the leg, supplies to the muscles and skin on top of the foot and adjacent sides of the first and second toe

111. Which nerve supplies impulses to the skin on the outer side and back of the foot and leg? (_____

    a) Saphenous

    b) Sural

    c) Dorsal

    d) Tibial

THE CIRCULATORY SYSTEM

112. The circulatory system, also referred to as the _____ or _____ system, controls the steady circulation of the blood through the body by means of the heart and blood vessels. It is made up of two divisions: the _____ , consisting of the _____ ; and the _____ _____ , which acts as an aid to the blood system and consists of the _____ , _____ and other structures.

113. The purpose of the blood vascular system is to _____ .

114. The purpose of lymph is to _____ .

115. Which of the following is referred to as the body's pump?

    ____ a) Cells

    ____ b) Lungs

    ____ c) Heart

    ____ d) Veins

116. Match the following chambers of the heart with their descriptions:

    ____ 1. Atrium   a) Structures between the chambers that allow the blood to flow in only one direction

    ____ 2. Ventricle   b) The upper, thin-walled chambers on the right and left

    ____ 3. Valves   c) The lower, thick-walled chambers on the right and left

117. Two systems circulate the blood constantly from the time it leaves the heart until it returns. They are _____ , which sends the blood from the heart to the lungs to be purified, and the _____ , which carries the blood from the heart throughout the body and back to the heart.

118. Explain how the pulmonary and systemic systems work:

a) _____

b) _____

c) _____

_____

d) _____

e) _____

f) _____

119. The three categories of blood vessels are _____ .

120. Match each of the following with its correct description:

____ 1. Arteries   a) Tiny, thin walled blood vessels that connect the smaller
                             arteries to the veins

____ 2. Capillaries   b) Thin walled blood vessels that are less elastic

____ 3. Veins   c) Thick walled, muscular, flexible tubes

121. Identify the anatomy of the heart illustrated:

To upper part of body

122. What is blood? _____

123. There are approximately _____ pints of blood in the human body, contributing to about _____ of the body's weight. Blood is approximately _____ water with a normal temperature of _____ °F.

124. Match each of the following with its correct description:

   ____ 1. Red blood cells   a) Contribute to the blood-clotting process

   ____ 2. Hemoglobin   b) The fluid part of the blood

   ____ 3. White blood cells   c) Produced in the red bone marrow

   ____ 4. Platelets   d) Perform the function of destroying disease-causing

                                      microorganisms

   ____ 5. Plasma   e) Complex iron protein that binds to oxygen

125. Blood performs the following critical functions:

a) _____

b) _____

_____

c) _____

_____

d) _____

e) _____

_____

126. The primary functions of the lymph vascular system are to:

a) _____

b) _____

c) _____

d) _____

127. The arteries that are located on either side of the neck and are the main sources of blood supply to the head, face and neck are the _____ arteries.

128. The internal carotid artery supplies blood to the _____
_____ .

129. The external carotid artery supplies blood to the _____
_____ .

130. The artery that supplies blood to the lower region of the face, mouth, and nose is the

_____.

    a) Facial artery

    b) Angular artery

    c) Superficial temporal artery

    d) Superior labial artery

131. The artery that supplies blood to the upper lip and region of the nose is the

_____.

    a) Facial artery

    b) Angular artery

    c) Superficial temporal artery

    d) Superior labial artery

132. The artery that supplies blood to the skin and masseter is the _____ .

    a) Parietal artery

    b) Transverse facial artery

    c) Middle temporal artery

    d) Anterior auricular artery

133. The popliteal artery divides into two separate arteries known as _____ .

    a) Parietal artery

    b) Transverse facial artery

    c) Middle temporal artery

    d) Anterior auricular artery

134. The _____ and _____ arteries are the main blood supply for the arms and hands.

135. Identify the arteries of the arm and hand illustrated:

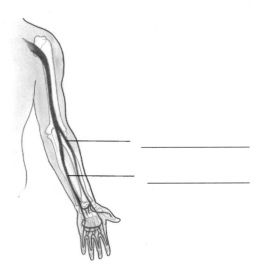

_____

_____

OTHER MAJOR SYSTEMS OF THE BODY

The endocrine system is made up of a group of specialized glands that affect:

    a) _____

    b) _____

    c) _____

    d) _____

136. What are glands? _____

_____

137. Name the two main types of glands and their functions:

    a) _____

    b) _____

       _____

138. The digestive system is responsible for: _____.

139. How long does the entire food digestion process take? _____

140. The _____ is responsible for purifying the body by eliminating waste.

141. Match each organ with its function in the excretory system:

   ____ 1. Kidneys   a) Eliminates decomposed and undigested food

   ____ 2. Liver   b) Eliminates waste containing perspiration

   ____ 3. Skin   c) Excrete waste containing urine

   ____ 4. Large intestine   d) Discharges waste containing bile

   ____ 5. Lungs   e) Exhale carbon dioxide

142. The respiratory system enables breathing or _____ and consists of the lungs and air passages.

143. The spongy tissues composed of microscopic cells in which inhaled air is exchanged for carbon dioxide during one breathing cycle are the _____ . The _____ is a muscular wall that separates the thorax from the abdominal region and helps control breathing.

144. During _____ or breathing in, oxygen is passed into the blood; during _____ or breathing outward, carbon dioxide is expelled from the lungs.

145. The _____ is made up of the skin and its various accessory organs such as the _____ , and _____ .

7 SKIN STRUCTURE & GROWTH

Date: _____

Rating: _____

Text Pages: 119-131

POINT TO PONDER

"To do a common thing uncommonly well brings success."
—Henry John Heinz

ANATOMY OF THE SKIN

1. The medical branch of science that deals with the study of skin and its nature, structure, functions, diseases, and treatment is called _____.

2. A _____ is a physician engaged in the science of treating the skin, its structures, functions, and diseases. An _____ is a specialist in the cleansing, preservation of health, and beautification of the skin and body.

3. The skin is the largest organ of the body.

   ____ True

   ____ False

4. The skin is our only barrier against the environment and protects

   a) _____

   b) _____

   c) _____

   d) _____

5. Healthy skin is _____.

6. The appendages of the skin include

   a) _____

   b) _____

   c) _____

   d) _____

7. The thinnest skin is found on the _____, and the thickest skin is found on the

   _____ .

8. Explain the difference between the skin of the scalp and the skin elsewhere on the
   human body. _____

   _____

9. The skin is composed of two main divisions, the _____ and the _____ .

10. The _____ is the outermost layer of the skin and is also called the _____ .
    It is the thinnest layer of skin and forms a _____ for the body.

11. The epidermis is made up of the following layers:

    a) _____

    b) _____

    c) _____

    d) _____

    e) _____

12. The basal cell layer is also referred to as the _____ and is the deepest
    layer of the epidermis. It is the _____ of the epidermis and is responsible for the
    growth of the _____ .

13. The basal cell layer also contains special cells called _____ , which produce
    a dark skin pigment called _____ .

14. The _____ also referred to as the stratum spinosum and is the layer that the
    beginning of the process that causes skin cells to shed begins.

15. The stratum granulosum, or _____ , consists of cells that are almost dead and
    are pushed to the surface to replace cells that are shed from the skin surface layer.

16. The _____ is the clear, transparent layer just under the skin surface, and
    the _____ is the outer layer of the epidermis.

17. Identify the layers of the skin illustrated below:

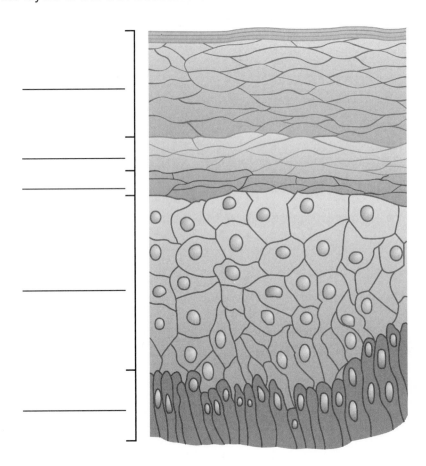

_____

_____

_____

_____

_____

18. The _____ is the underlying or inner layer of the skin and is made up of two layers: the _____ and the _____.

19. Which layer is the outer layer of the dermis, located directly beneath the epidermis?

_____

20. Which layer is the deeper layer of the dermis that supplies the skin with oxygen and nutrients? _____

21. The reticular layer contains the following structures within its network:

a) _____

b) _____

c) _____

d) _____

e) _____

f) _____

g) _____

22. Where is the subcutaneous or fatty layer found? _____

23. This fatty tissue is also called _____ or _____ tissue and varies in thickness according to _____ , and _____

24. _____ supplies nutrients and oxygen to the skin. _____ , the clear fluids of the body that resemble blood plasma, bathe the skin cells, _____ and _____ , and have immune functions that help protect the skin and body against diseases.

25. The skin contains the surface endings of the following nerve fibers:

    a) _____

    b) _____

    c) _____

26. _____ nerve fibers react to heat, cold, touch, pressure, and pain.

27. _____ nerve fibers are distributed to the arrector pili muscles.

28. Which nerve fibers are part of the autonomic nervous system, regulate the excretion of perspiration from the sweat glands, and control the flow of sebum? _____

29. The nerve endings that provide the body with the sense of touch are housed in the _____ layer of the dermis.

30. The color of the skin depends primarily on _____ , which are tiny grains of pigment deposited into cells in the _____ of the epidermis and papillary layers of the dermis.

31. Name and describe the two types of melanin:

    a) _____

    b) _____

32. What are the two structures that skin gets its strength, form, and flexibility from?

    a) _____

    b) _____

33. The skin contains two types of duct glands, _____ and _____ , that extract materials from the blood to form new substances.

34. The sudoriferous glands excrete

　　＿＿ a) Fragrance

　　＿＿ b) Water

　　＿＿ c) Oil

　　＿＿ d) Sweat

35. The sweat glands regulate ＿＿＿＿＿＿＿＿＿＿＿ and help to eliminate ＿＿＿＿＿＿＿＿ ＿＿＿＿＿＿＿＿ from the body. The are found on all parts of the body but are more numerous on the ＿＿＿＿＿＿＿＿＿＿＿＿＿＿＿＿＿＿＿＿＿＿＿＿＿ .

36. The excretion of sweat is controlled by the ＿＿＿＿＿＿＿＿＿ and normally, ＿＿＿＿＿＿＿＿＿＿＿ of liquids containing salts are eliminated daily through sweat pores.

37. The sebaceous or oil glands of the skin are connected to the ＿＿＿＿＿＿＿＿＿＿＿＿ .

38. ＿＿＿＿＿＿＿ is a fatty or oil secretion that lubricates the skin and preserves the softness of the hair.

39. Sebaceous glands are not found on the

　　＿＿ a) Scalp

　　＿＿ b) Palms

　　＿＿ c) Face

　　＿＿ d) Knees

40. When the sebum hardens and the duct becomes clogged, a pore impaction or ＿＿＿＿＿＿ is formed.

41. List the principle functions of the skin:

a) ＿＿＿＿＿＿＿＿＿＿＿＿＿＿＿＿＿＿＿＿＿＿＿＿＿＿＿＿＿＿＿＿＿＿＿＿

b) ＿＿＿＿＿＿＿＿＿＿＿＿＿＿＿＿＿＿＿＿＿＿＿＿＿＿＿＿＿＿＿＿＿＿＿＿

c) ＿＿＿＿＿＿＿＿＿＿＿＿＿＿＿＿＿＿＿＿＿＿＿＿＿＿＿＿＿＿＿＿＿＿＿＿

d) ＿＿＿＿＿＿＿＿＿＿＿＿＿＿＿＿＿＿＿＿＿＿＿＿＿＿＿＿＿＿＿＿＿＿＿＿

e) ＿＿＿＿＿＿＿＿＿＿＿＿＿＿＿＿＿＿＿＿＿＿＿＿＿＿＿＿＿＿＿＿＿＿＿＿

f) ＿＿＿＿＿＿＿＿＿＿＿＿＿＿＿＿＿＿＿＿＿＿＿＿＿＿＿＿＿＿＿＿＿＿＿＿

MAINTAINING THE HEALTH OF THE SKIN

42. The best way to support the health of the skin is to ＿＿＿＿＿＿＿＿＿＿＿＿＿＿＿＿ ＿＿＿＿＿＿＿＿＿＿＿＿＿＿＿＿＿＿＿＿＿＿＿＿＿＿＿＿＿＿＿＿ .

43. Match the following vitamin with its effect on healthy skin:

___ 1. Vitamin A   a) Promotes the healthy and rapid healing of skin

___ 2. Vitamin C   b) Aids in the health, function, and repair of skin cells

___ 3. Vitamin D   c) Helps heal damage to the skin's tissues when used both
                          internally and externally

___ 4. Vitamin E   d) Aids in and speeds up the healing process of the body

44. Water comprises _____ of the body's weight.

45. Drinking pure water is essential to the health of the skin and body because it

a) _____

b) _____

c) _____

d) _____

46. Explain how to determine the amount of water needed every day for maximum physical
health. _____

_____

8 NAIL STRUCTURE & GROWTH

Date: _____

Rating: _____

Text Pages: 132-138

POINT TO PONDER:

> *"He who is afraid of doing too much always does too little."*
> *—German Proverb*

1. The _____ is a hard, protective plate made of a protein called _____.

2. The keratin found in the natural nail is not as hard as the keratin found in the hair or skin.

   ___ a) True

   ___ b) False

3. Describe the appearance of a healthy nail: _____

   _____

4. The nail plate is relatively _____ to water, allowing water to pass more easily than it will pass through normal skin of equal thickness.

5. The nail may look dry and hard, but is actually has a water content of between _____ water, which varies based on the relative humidity of the surrounding environment.

   a) 5% and 10%

   b) 10% and 20%

   c) 15% and 25%

   d) 20% and 30%

6. Water directly affects the nail's _____ The lower the water content, the more

   _____ .

7. What can be done to reduce water loss and improve flexibility? _____

   _____

8. Identify the parts of the nail as illustrated below:

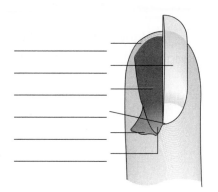   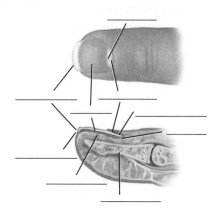

9. The _____ is the portion of living skin on which the nail plate sits.

10. The nail bed is supplied with many nerves and is attached to the nail plate by a thin layer of tissue called the _____ .

11. The _____ is where the natural nail is formed.

12. The visible part of the matrix that extends from underneath the living skin is called the

_____

13. Growth of the nails can be affected if an individual is in

a) _____

b) _____

c) _____

14. The _____ is the most visible and functional part of the nail module. It is constructed of about _____ layers of nail cells.

15. The part of the nail plate that extends over the tip of the finger or toe is the _____ .

16. The _____ is the dead, colorless tissue attached to the nail plate.

17. What is the purpose of the cuticle? _____

_____

_____

18. The living skin at the base of the nail plate covering the matrix area is the _____ .

19. Describe the difference between the eponychium and the cuticle: _____

_____

20. The _____ is the slightly thickened layer of skin that lies underneath the free edge of the nail plate.

21. A tough band of fibrous tissue that connects bones or holds an organ in place is a

_____ .

22. Specialized ligaments attach the nail bed and _____ to the underlying bone and are located at the base of the matrix and around the edges of the nail bed.

23. The _____ are folds of normal skin that surround the nail plate which forms nail grooves.

24. What are nail grooves? _____

_____

NAIL GROWTH

25. The growth of the nail plate is affected by _____ .

26. Identify the various shapes of nails in the illustration below:

27. The average rate of nail growth in the normal adult is:

____ a) ½" per month

____ b) ½" per week

____ c) ¹⁄₁₀" per month

____ d) ⅛" per week

28. Nails grow faster in the winter than they do in the summer.

____ True

____ False

29. Children's nails grow more rapidly; elderly persons grow at a slower rate.

____ True

____ False

30. The nail of the middle finger grows fastest and the thumbnail grows the slowest.

____ True

____ False

31. What causes the growth rates of the nail to increase dramatically during pregnancy?

_____

32. What will cause the shape or thickness of the nail plate to change? _____

_____

33. How long does replacement of the natural nail take? _____

34. Toenails take _____ months to be fully replaced.

a) 3

b) 5

c) 7

d) 9

35. Like hair, the nail will automatically shed periodically.

____ True

____ False

9 PROPERTIES OF THE HAIR & SCALP

Date: _____

Rating: _____

Text Pages: 139-163

POINT TO PONDER:

"Never give up then, for it is just the place and time that the tide will turn."
—*Harriet Beecher Stow*

STRUCTURE OF THE HAIR

1. _____ is the scientific study of hair, its diseases, and care, which comes from the Greek words _____ meaning hair and _____ meaning "the study of."

2. The hair, skin, and nails is collectively know as the _____.

3. A mature strand of human hair is divided into two parts: the _____ located below the surface of the scalp, and the _____ the portion of the hair that projects above the skin.

4. Match the main structure of the hair root with their description:

   ___ 1. Follicle   a) Small, cone-shaped area located at the base of the follicle

   ___ 2. Bulb   b) The tube-like depression in the skin or scalp that contains the hair root

   ___ 3. Dermal papilla   c) Involuntary muscle in the base of the hair follicle

   ___ 4. Arrector pili   d) The oil glands of the skin

   ___ 5. Sebaceous glands   e) Thickened, club-shaped structure; forms the lower part of the root

5. Hair follicles are distributed all over the body, with the exception of

   a) _____

   b) _____

6. Which part of the root contains the blood and nerve supply that provides the nutrients needed for hair growth? _____

7. Which muscle when contracted causes goose bumps? _____

8. The sebaceous glands secrete an oily substance called _____ , which lubricates the hair and skin.

9. Identify the parts of the skin and hair illustrated below:

10. What are the three main layers of the hair shaft?

   a) _____

   b) _____

   c) _____

11. The outermost layer of the hair is the _____ .

12. Describe the cuticle layer: _____
   _____

13. Describe what a healthy cuticle layer protects: _____
   _____

14. Why must oxidation haircolors, permanent waving solutions, and chemical hair relaxers have an alkaline pH? _____
   _____

15. Which layer of the hair is the cortex? _____

16. What percentage of weight of the hair comes from the cortex?

____ a) 50%

____ b) 70%

____ c) 80%

____ d) 90%

17. In what layer of the hair do changes involving oxidation haircolor, wet setting, thermal styling, permanent waving, and chemical hair relaxing take place? _____

18. The _____ is the innermost layer of the hair and is composed of round cells.

19. All hair has three layers—the cuticle, the cortex, and the medulla.

____ True

____ False

20. Identify the cross-section of the hair as illustrated below:

THE CHEMICAL COMPOSITION OF HAIR

21. Hair is composed of _____ that grows from cells originating within the hair follicle.

22. The maturation of these cells is a process called _____.

23. Hair is a living thing.

____ True

____ False

Explain your answer: _____

_____

24. List the main elements that make up human hair and their percentages in normal hair:

a) _____

b) _____

c) _____

d) _____

e) _____

25. Match the following terms with their description:

_____ 1. Amino acid   a) The chemical bond that links amino acids

_____ 2. Helix   b) The unit of structure that build proteins

_____ 3. Peptide bond   c) A long chain of amino acids linked by peptide bonds

_____ 4. Polypeptide chain   d) The spiral shape of a coiled protein

26. Polypeptide chains are cross-linked together using three different types of cross links called:

a) _____

b) _____

c) _____

27. A _____ bond is a weak physical side bond that is easily broken by water or heat.

28. Weak, temporary side bonds between adjacent polypeptide chains are _____ bonds.

29. A _____ bond is a strong chemical side bond that joins the sulfur atom of two neighboring cysteine amino acids to create cystine.

30. What layer of the hair is all natural color located in? _____

31. _____ are the tiny grains of pigment that give natural color to the hair. There are two different types. List and describe

a) _____

b) _____

32. The _____ of the hair refers to the shape of the hair strand and is described as _____ or _____

33. Natural wave patterns are the result of _____

34. In extremely curly hair, cross-sections are highly _____ and vary in shape and thickness along their length.

HAIR ANALYSIS

35. List and define the four most important factors to consider in hair analysis

    a) _____

    b) _____

    c) _____

    _____

    d) _____

36. What is the classification of hair texture?

    a) _____

    b) _____

    c) _____

37. Does all hair on a persons head have the same texture?

    ____ Yes

    ____ No

38. Which hair texture has the largest diameter? _____

39. Which hair texture is the most common and is the standard? _____

40. Which hair texture has the smallest diameter and is more fragile? _____

41. Hair density can be classified as

    a) _____

    b) _____

    c) _____

42. The average hair density is about _____ hairs per square inch, and the average head of hair contains about _____ individual hair strands.

43. The hair's ability to absorb moisture is its _____

44. The degree of porosity is directly related to _____ Why?

    _____

    _____

45. Chemical services performed on overly porous hair require _____ .

46. Hair with average porosity is considered _____ . Overly porous hair is _____
_____ .

47. Describe how to check porosity: _____
_____
_____

48. If it feels smooth, _____ .

49. If you can feel a slight roughness, _____ .

50. If the hair feels very rough or dry or breaks, _____
_____ .

51. The ability of the hair to stretch and return to its original length without breaking is its
_____ .

52. Hair elasticity is an indication of _____
_____ .

53. Wet hair with normal elasticity will stretch up to _____ of its original length and
return without breaking. Dry hair stretches about _____ of its length.

54. Hair follicles always grow perpendicular (90-degree angle) to the scalp.

   ____ True
   ____ False

55. Match the following terms with their description:

   ____ 1. Hair stream   a) Hair following in the same direction
   ____ 2. Whorl   b) A tuft of hair that stands straight up
   ____ 3. Cowlick   c) Hair that forms in a circular patter

56. Which of the following is not a cause of dry hair and scalp?

   ____ a) Winter weather
   ____ b) Desert climate
   ____ c) Inactive sebaceous glands
   ____ d) Active sebaceous glands

57. Oily hair and scalp is caused by _____ or _____ sebaceous glands and is characterized by a greasy buildup on the scalp and an oily coating on the hair.

58. Dry hair and scalp can be caused by inactive _____ and is aggravated by excessive _____ .

59. Oily hair and scalp is characterized by _____

_____ .

HAIR GROWTH

60. The two main types of hair found on the body are _____ and _____ hair.

61. Describe vellus hair: _____

_____

62. On adults, vellus hair is usually found on the _____ .

63. Describe terminal hair: _____

_____

64. Terminal hair is found on the _____ .

65. Unscramble these words, then match them with their correct description:

gloeten   neanag   agatecn

_____   The growth phase of new hair

_____   The transition phase

_____   The resting phase

66. What is the average growth of healthy scalp hair per month?

____ a) ¼"
____ b) ½"
____ c) ¾"
____ d) 1"

67. What percentage of scalp hair is in the catagen phase at any one time?

____ a) 1%
____ b) 5%
____ c) 10%
____ d) 15%

68. What percentage of scalp hair is in the telogen phase at any one time?

___ a) 1%

___ b) 5%

___ c) 10%

___ d) 15%

69. Shaving, clipping, and cutting the hair makes it grow back faster, darker, and coarser.

___ True

___ False

70. Scalp massage increases hair growth.

___ True

___ False

71. Gray hair is coarser and more resistant than pigmented hair.

___ True

___ False

HAIR LOSS

72. It is normal to lose some hair every day.

___ True

___ False

73. Abnormal hair loss is called _____ .

74. _____ or androgenetic alopecia is the result of genetics, age, and hormonal changes that cause miniaturization of terminal hair, converting it to _____ hair.

75. In men, androgenic alopecia is known as _____ and usually progresses to the familiar horseshoe-shaped fringe of hair.

76. How many people does androgenic alopecia affect in the United States? _____

_____

77. _____ is characterized by the sudden falling out of hair in round patches or baldness in spots and may occur on the scalp and elsewhere on the body.

78. What is alopecia areata? _____

_____

_____

79. A temporary hair loss experienced at the conclusion of a pregnancy is _____

_____.

80. What are the only two products that have been proven to stimulate hair growth and are approved by the Food and Drug Administration (FDA)? _____

81. A topical medication that is applied to the scalp twice a day, and is sold over-the-counter as a nonprescription drug is _____

82. _____ is an oral prescription medication for men only and is more effective and convenient than minoxidil.

83. Describe surgical treatments for hair loss:

_____

_____

84. What nonmedical options can a hairstylist offer to counter hair loss? _____

_____

DISORDERS OF THE HAIR

85. Match the following hair disorders with its description:

___ 1. Canities	a) A condition of abnormal growth of hair
___ 2. Ringed hair	b) Technical term for gray hair
___ 3. Hypertrichosis	c) Knotted hair
___ 4. Trichoptilosis	d) Technical term for beaded hair
___ 5. Trichorrhexis nodosa	e) Technical term for brittle hair
___ 6. Monilethrix	f) Characterized by alternating bands of gray and pigmented hair
___ 7. Fragilitas crinium	g) Technical term for split ends

86. There are two types of canities: they are _____ and _____

87. What is an example of hypertrichosis? _____. What are possible treatments? _____

_____

DISORDERS OF THE SCALP

88. What is the difference between dry scalp and dandruff? _____

_____

_____

89. Match the following scalp disorders with its definition:

___ 1. Pityriasis	a) Medical term for ringworm
___ 2. Tinea	b) Dry, sulfur-yellow, cup-like crusts on the scalp called scutula
___ 3. Tinea capitis	c) An acute, localized bacterial infection of the hair follicle
___ 4. Tinea favosa	d) Medical term for dandruff
___ 5. Scabies	e) An inflammation of the subcutaneous tissue caused by staphylococci
___ 6. Pediculosis capitis	f) Fungal infection characterized by red papules, or spots at the opening of the hair follicles
___ 7. Furuncle	g) The infestation of the hair and scalp with head lice
___ 8. Carbuncle	h) Caused by a parasite called a "mite"

90. Research confirms that dandruff is the result of a fungus called _____ , a naturally occurring fungus that is present on all human skin.

91. What is the treatment for dandruff? _____

_____

92. List the two principle types of dandruff and give their characterizations:

a) _____

_____

b) _____

_____

93. What does tinea look like? _____

_____

94. Is tinea contagious?

___ Yes

___ No

10 BASICS OF CHEMISTRY

Date: _____

Rating: _____

Text Pages: 164-178

POINT TO PONDER:

"Success seems to be connected with action. Successful people keep moving. They make mistakes, but they don't quit."—**Conrad Hilton**

CHEMISTRY

1. _____ is the science that deals with the composition, structures, and properties of matter and how matter changes under different conditions.

2. _____ is the study of substances that contain carbon.

3. The term "organic" does not mean "natural."

   ___ True

   ___ False

MATTER

4. _____ is the study of substances that do not contain carbon.

5. Match each of the following with its correct description:

   ___ 1. Matter   a) The simplest form of matter

   ___ 2. Elements   b) A chemical combination of two or more atoms

   ___ 3. Atoms   c) Any substance that occupies space and has mass

   ___ 4. Molecule   d) The particles from which all matter is composed

6. All matter has physical and chemical properties and exists in the form of _____ or _____ .

7. _____ does not occupy space or have mass.

8. There are _____ naturally occurring elements, each with its own distinct physical and chemical properties.

9. An _____ is the smallest particle of an element that retains the properties of that element.

10. _____ are a chemical combination of atoms of the same element.

11. _____ are chemical combinations of two or more atoms of different elements.

12. _____ are the three different physical forms of matter.

13. Match the three different states of matter with their corresponding characteristics:

    ____ 1. Solids   a) Do not have a definite shape or volume

    ____ 2. Liquids   b) Have a definite shape and volume

    ____ 3. Gases   c) Have a definite volume but not a definite shape

14. _____ are those characteristics that can be determined without a chemical reaction and do not include a chemical change. Physical properties include

_____ .

15. _____ are those characteristics that can only be determined by a chemical reaction and a chemical change in the substance. List two examples: _____

_____

16. What is oxidation? _____

_____

17. A change in the form or physical properties of a substance without a chemical reaction or the creation of a new substance is a _____ .

18. What are two examples of a physical change?

    a) _____

    b) _____

19. A change in the chemical and physical properties of a substance by a chemical reaction is a _____ .

20. List two examples of a chemical change:

    a) _____

    b) _____

21. A _____ is a chemical combination of matter, in definite proportions.

22. What are some examples of a pure substance? _____

23. A physical mixture is a physical combination of _____ in any proportions.

24. Match the following with their description:

    ___ 1. Solution   a) A stable mixture of two or more mixable substances

    ___ 2. Solute   b) The substance that dissolves

    ___ 3. Solvent   c) The substance that is dissolved

25. _____ liquids are mutually soluble, meaning that they can be mixed into stable solutions.

26. _____ liquids are not capable of being mixed into stable solutions.

27. An unstable mixture of undissolved particles in a liquid is a

    ___ a) Emulsion

    ___ b) Suspension

    ___ c) Surfactant

28. An unstable mixture of two or more immiscible substances united with the aid of an emulsifier is an

    ___ a) Emulsion

    ___ b) Suspension

    ___ c) Surfactant

29. Substances that act as a bridge to allow oil and water to mix or emulsify are

    ___ a) Emulsion

    ___ b) Suspension

    ___ c) Surfactants

30. An example of a suspension is _____ .

31. A surfactant molecule has two distinct parts. The head is _____ , meaning water-loving, and the tail is _____ , meaning oil-loving.

32. An example of an oil-in-water emulsion is _____ Describe why: _____

    _____

    _____

33. What are two examples of a water-in-oil emulsion? _____

34. Isopropyl alcohol and ethyl alcohol are both _____ alcohols.

35. Match the following chemical ingredients with their description:

    ____ 1. Alkonolamines   a) A special type of oil used in hair conditioners

    ____ 2. Ammonia   b) Sweet, colorless, oily substance

    ____ 3. Glycerine   c) Substances used to neutralize acids or raise

                                the pH of many hair products

    ____ 4. Silicones   d) Contain carbon and evaporate quickly

    ____ 5. Volatile organic compounds   e) A colorless gas with a pungent odor

POTENTIAL HYDROGEN

36. What does pH stand for? _____

37. An _____ is an atom or molecule that carries an electrical charge. _____ causes an atom or molecule to split in two, creating a pair of ions with opposite electrical charges.

38. An ion with a negative electrical charge is an _____ an ion with a positive electrical charge is a _____ .

39. What does the pH scale measure? _____

40. The pH scale ranges from 0 to 14. Match the following pH values with their description:

    ____ 1. pH below 7   a) A neutral solution

    ____ 2. pH of 7   b) An acidic solution

    ____ 3. pH above 7   c) An alkaline solution

41. The term _____ means multiples of 10.

42. All _____ owe their chemical reactivity to the hydrogen ion. Acids have a pH below _____ and turn litmus paper from _____ Acids _____ and _____ the hair.

43. All _____ owe their chemical reactivity to the hydroxide ion. The term _____ and _____ are interchangeable. Alkalis have a pH above _____ and turn litmus paper from _____ . Alkalis _____ and _____ the hair and skin.

44. Neutralizing shampoos and normalizing lotions used to neutralize hydroxide hair relaxers work by creating an acid-alkali _____ reaction.

45. _____ reactions are responsible for the chemical changes created by hair colors, hair lighteners, permanent wave solutions, and neutralizers.

46. _____ is a chemical reaction that combines a substance with oxygen to produce an oxide.

47. Chemical reactions that produce heat are called _____ .

48. _____ is the rapid oxidation of substance, accompanied by the production of heat and light.

49. Provide the description for the following terms:

    a) Oxidized   _____

    b) Reduced   _____

    c) Reduction   _____

                               _____

    d) Oxidizing agent   _____

50. What is an example of an oxidizing agent? _____

51. Oxidation and reduction reactions always occur at the same time and are referred to as _____ and involve a transfer between the _____ and the

_____.

52. Oxidation is the result of either the addition of _____ or the _____ of hydrogen.

11 BASICS OF ELECTRICITY

Date: _____

Rating: _____

Text Pages: 179-192

POINT TO PONDER:

"Success is going from failure to failure without losing your enthusiasm."
—Abraham Lincoln

ELECTRICITY

1. _____ is a form of energy; it is a flow of negatively charged _____ .

2. An _____ is a flow of electricity along a conductor.

3. Any substance that easily transmits electricity is a _____ .

4. Which of the following is a conductor?

    ____ a) Wood

    ____ b) Copper

    ____ c) Cloth

    ____ d) Alcohol

5. A substance that does not easily transmit electricity is an _____ or a _____ .

6. Which of the following is not an insulator?

    ____ a) Rubber

    ____ b) Silk

    ____ c) Cement

    ____ d) Water

7. A _____ is the path of an electric current from the generating source through the conductor and back to its original source.

8. Name the two types of electric current:

   a) _____

   b) _____

9. Direct current, is an constant, even-flowing current that travels in _____ direction and is produced by _____ .

10. _____ current is a rapid and interrupted current, flowing first in one direction and then in the opposite direction.

11. What apparatus changes direct current to alternating current? _____

12. What apparatus changes alternating current to direct current? _____

13. Match the following words with their correct definitions:

   ____ 1. Volt   a) Measures the strength of an electrical current

   ____ 2. Amp   b) Measures how much electric energy is used in one second

   ____ 3. Milliampere   c) Is 1,000 watts

   ____ 4. Ohm   d) Measures the pressure or force that pushes the flow of
                            electrons through a conductor

   ____ 5. Watt   e) Is 1/1000th of an ampere

   ____ 6. Kilowatt   f) Measures the resistance of an electric current

14. A device that prevents excessive current from passing through a circuit is a _____ .

15. A switch that automatically interrupts or shuts off an electric circuit at the first indication of overload is a _____ .

16. List all of the safety guidelines that you should adhere to when using electric appliances in the salon:

   a) _____

   b) _____

   c) _____

   d) _____

   e) _____

   f) _____

   _____

g) _____

_____

h) _____

i) _____

_____

j) _____

k) _____

_____

l) _____

m) _____

n) _____

o) _____

ELECTROTHERAPY

17. _____ are commonly referred to as electrotherapy.

18. A _____ or _____ is an instrument that plugs into an ordinary wall outlet and produces different types of electric currents that are used for _____ _____ They are called _____ .

19. An _____ is an applicator for directing the electric current from the machine to the client's skin and is usually made of _____ or _____ .

20. _____ indicates the negative and positive poles of an electric current. Electrotherapy devices always have one negatively charged pole, called an _____ and one positively charged pole, called an _____ .

21. The positive electrode is usually _____ and is marked with a "P" or a plus (+) sign.

22. The negative electrode is usually _____ and is marked with an "N" or minus (−) sign.

23. Explain how to determine the polarity if the electrodes are not marked:

a) _____

_____

_____

_____

b) _____

_____

_____

24. List the two modalities used in cosmetology:

a) _____

b) _____

25. Which one is the most commonly used modality? _____

26. The electrode used on the area to be treated is the _____ electrode; the _____ electrode is the opposite pole.

27. _____ is the process of introducing water-soluble products into the skin with the use of electric current.

28. _____ forces acidic substances into deeper tissues using galvanic current from the positive toward the negative pole.

29. _____ is the process of forcing liquids into the tissues from the negative toward the positive pole.

30. _____ is a process used to soften and emulsify grease deposits and blackheads in the hair follicles.

31. The _____ is a thermal or heat-producing current with a high frequency, commonly called the _____ and is used for both scalp and facial treatments.

32. The Tesla current electrodes are made from either _____ or _____ .

33 List the benefits from the use of Tesla high-frequency current:

a) _____

b) _____

c) _____

d) _____

e) _____

f) _____

OTHER ELECTRICAL EQUIPMENT

34. List the use or description of the following electrical equipment:

a) Hood hair dryers/heat lamps

_____

_____

b) Curling and flat irons

_____

_____

c) Heating cap

_____

_____

d) Haircolor processing machines

_____

_____

_____

e) Steamer or vaporizer

_____

_____

LIGHT THERAPY

35. _____ is electromagnetic radiation that we can see. Electromagnetic radiation is also called _____ because it carries energy through space on waves.

36. The distance between two successive peaks is called the _____. Long wavelengths have low frequency, meaning _____ within a given length. Short wavelengths have higher frequency, meaning _____ within a given length.

37. The entire range of wavelengths of electromagnetic radiation is called the

_____ .

38. Visible light makes up _____ of natural sunlight.

39. _____ and _____ are invisible because their wavelengths are beyond the visible spectrum of light. They make up _____ of natural sunlight.

40. _____ have long wavelengths, penetrate the deepest, and produce the most heat.

41. At what distance and for how long should infrared lamps be used during hair treatments?

_____

42. _____ are the primary source of lights used for facial and scalp treatments.

43. The bulbs used for therapeutic visible light therapy are _____ and _____.

44. _____ is referred to as _____ because it is a combination of all the visible rays of the spectrum.

45. The benefit of white light is that _____

_____.

46. Blue light should only be used on _____ that is bare.

47. The benefit of blue light is that _____

_____.

48. Red light is used on _____ in combination with oils and creams.

49. The benefit of red light is that _____.

50. _____ make up 5% of natural sunlight and are referred to as _____

or _____.

51. Ultraviolet rays are applied with a lamp at a distance of _____ with an exposure times of _____ Times may be gradually increased to

_____.

52. _____ are used to make reactions happen more quickly. They may be either a _____ energy source or a _____ source.

12 PRINCIPLES OF HAIR DESIGN

Date: _____

Rating: _____

Text Pages: 194-216

POINT TO PONDER:

> *"A year from now you may wish you had started today."*—*Karen Lamb*

PHILOSOPHY OF DESIGN
_____

1. When designing a hairstyle for your client, what is your goal? _____

    _____

2. What should a good designer always visualize before beginning? _____

3. List some sources of inspiration: _____

    _____

4. What places, things, or people inspire your creativity? _____

    _____

5. Once you have been inspired, what is the next step? _____

    _____

6. As a designer, what must you develop? _____

    _____

7. This can not be achieved through book-learning, the best teacher is _____

    _____ .

8. Having a strong foundation in technique and skills will allow you to take _____

    _____ .

9. What does it mean to "think out of the box"? _____

    _____

    _____

    _____

ELEMENTS OF HAIR DESIGN

10. What are the five basic elements of three dimensional design:

a) _____

b) _____

c) _____

d) _____

e) _____

11. _____ create the shape, design and movement of a hairstyle. They can be _____

or _____ .

12. Match the four basic types of lines with their descriptions:

____ 1. Horizontal lines   a) Lines are up and down

____ 2. Vertical lines   b) Large or small, a full circle or just part of a circle

____ 3. Diagonal lines   c) Positioned between horizontal and vertical lines

____ 4. Curved lines   d) Extend in the same direction and maintain

         a constant distance apart

13. Describe the usage of the basic types of lines:

a) Horizontal lines: _____

b) Vertical lines: _____

c) Diagonal lines: _____

d) Curved lines: _____

14. Describe a single-line in hairstyling: _____

_____

15. Describe a parallel line in hairstyling: _____

_____

16. Describe a contrasting line in hairstyling: _____

_____

17. Describe a transitional line in hairstyling: _____

_____

18. _____ is a mass or general outline of a hairstyle that is three-dimensional and has

_____ , and _____ .

19. Form or mass may also be called _____ .

20. The _____ is usually the part of the overall design that a client will respond to first.

21. The hair form should be in proportion to the shape of the

    a) _____

    b) _____

    c) _____

22. _____ is the area surrounding the form or the area the hairstyle occupies and may contain _____ , or any combination.

23. Wave patterns or _____ must be taken into consideration when designing a style for a client.

24. All hair has a natural wave pattern described as

    a) _____

    b) _____

    c) _____

    d) _____

25. How can texture be created temporarily? _____

_____

26. How can texture be changed permanently? _____

27. When is it appropriate to use many wave pattern combinations together? _____

_____

_____

28. _____ wave patterns accent the face and are useful when you wish to narrow a round head shape.

29. _____ wave patterns take attention away from the face and can be used to soften square or rectangular features.

30. What two roles does color play in hair design?

    a) _____

    b) _____

31. _____ can be used to make all or part of the design appear larger or smaller and can help define _____ and _____ .

32. Light colors and warm colors create the illusion of _____ .

33. _____ and _____ colors recede or move in toward the head, creating the illusion of less volume.

34. Explain how to create the illusion of dimension or depth: _____

    _____

35. Using a _____ color will draw a line in the hairstyle in the direction you want the eye to travel.

36. What should be considered when choosing a color? _____

    _____

PRINCIPLES OF HAIR DESIGN
_____

37. The five principles for art and design of hair design are

    a) _____

    b) _____

    c) _____

    d) _____

    e) _____

38. Match the following principle of design with its description:

    ____ 1. Proportion   a) Where the eye is drawn to first

    ____ 2. Balance   b) Creation of unity

    ____ 3. Rhythm   c) Establishing equal or appropriate proportions to
                                   create symmetry

    ____ 4. Emphasis   d) Regular pulsation or recurrent pattern of
                                   movement in a design

    ____ 5. Harmony   e) The comparative relationship of one thing to another.

39. It is essential when designing a hairstyle that you take into account the client's _____

    _____ .

40. What style would you normally create for a woman with large hips or broad shoulders?

    _____

41. What is the general guide for "classic" proportion? _____
_____

42. Which element of design can be either symmetrical or asymmetrical? _____

43. Explain how to measure symmetry: _____
_____

44. Describe symmetrical balance: _____
_____
_____
_____

45. Describe asymmetrical balance: _____
_____
_____

46. Which of the following signifies a fast rhythm?

____ a) Tight curls

____ b) Loose curls

47. Create interest in a hairstyle with an area of focus or emphasis by using

a) _____

b) _____

c) _____

d) _____

48. Which element of design holds all the elements of the design together? _____

49. The best results are obtained when your client's facial features are properly analyzed for their _____ and _____ .

50. An artistic and suitable hairstyle will take into account the following characteristics of the client:

a) _____

b) _____

c) _____

INFLUENCE OF HAIR TYPE ON HAIRSTYLE

51. Hair type is a major consideration in the selection of a hairstyle. What are the two main characterizations to consider? _____

52. Match each of the following hair textures with its description:

_____ 1. Fine, straight hair   a) Offers the most versatility in styling

_____ 2. Straight, medium hair   b) Hard to curl; responds well to thermal styling

_____ 3. Straight coarse hair   c) Often separates, revealing the client's scalp

_____ 4. Wavy, fine hair   d) Generally best left short

_____ 5. Wavy, medium hair   e) When left natural gives a soft romantic look

_____ 6. Wavy, coarse hair   f) Can get very wide, rather than longer, as it
                                               grows

_____ 7. Curly, fine hair   g) Hugs the head shape because of no body
                                               or volume

_____ 8. Curly, medium hair   h) May appear fuller with appropriate haircut
                                               and style; hair can be fragile

_____ 9. Curly, coarse hair   i) Will be extremely wide without proper
                                               maintenance

_____ 10. Very curly, fine hair   j) Needs heavy styling products to weight
                                               it down

_____ 11. Extremely curly, medium hair   k) Hair could appear unruly if it is not shaped
                                               properly

_____ 12. Extremely curly, coarse hair   l) Offers more versatility; good amount of
                                               movement

FACIAL TYPES

53. A client's facial shape is determined by the _____ and _____ of the facial bones.

54. List the seven basic facial shapes:

a) _____

b) _____

c) _____

d) _____

e) _____

f) _____

g) _____

55. When designing a style for your client's facial type, you generally are trying to create the illusion of an _____-shaped face.

56. To determine a facial shape, divide the face into _____ zones. They are _____

_____.

57. Describe the facial contour of the oval face: _____

_____

58. Describe the facial contour, the aim, and the styling choice for the round-shaped face:

Contour: _____

Aim: _____

Styling choice: _____

_____

59. Describe the facial contour, the aim, and the styling choice for the square-shaped face:

Contour: _____

_____

Aim: _____

Styling choice: _____

_____

60. Describe the facial contour, the aim, and the styling choice for the triangular-shaped (pear-shaped) face:

Contour: _____

Aim: _____

Styling choice: _____

61. Describe the facial contour, the aim, and the styling choice for the oblong-shaped face:

Contour: _____

Aim: _____

Styling choice: _____

_____

62. Describe the facial contour, the aim, and the styling choice for the diamond-shaped face:

Contour: _____

Aim: _____

Styling choice: _____

_____

63. Describe the facial contour, the aim, and the styling choice for the inverted triangle-shaped (heart-shaped) face:

Contour: _____

Aim: _____

_____

Styling choice: _____

_____

64. The _____ is the outline of the face, head or figure seen in a side view.

65. Match the following basic profiles with their descriptions:

____ 1. Straight   a) Has a prominent forehead and chin

____ 2. Convex   b) Considered ideal; has slight curvature

____ 3. Concave   c) Has receding forehead and chin

66. How should you style the hair for a wide forehead? _____

_____

67. How should you style the hair for a narrow forehead? _____

_____

68. How should you style the hair for close-set eyes? _____

_____

69. How should you style the hair for wide-set eyes? _____

_____

70. How should you style the hair for a crooked nose? _____

71. How should you style the hair for a wide, flat nose? _____

_____

72. How should you style the hair for a long, narrow nose? _____

_____

73. Provide the correct styling aid for the following facial features:

    a) Round jaw _____

    b) Square jaw _____

    c) Long jaw _____

    d) Receding forehead _____

       _____

    e) Large forehead _____

    f) Small nose _____

    g) Prominent nose _____

    h) Receding chin _____

    i) Small chin _____

    j) Large chin _____

74. How should you style the hair for a head that is not completely round? _____

    _____

    _____

75. What is a major consideration when creating a hairstyle for someone who wears glasses?

    _____

    _____

76. List the three ways that the bang area or fringe can be parted:

    a) _____

    b) _____

    c) _____

77. List the four parts that can be used to highlight facial features:

    a) _____

    b) _____

    c) _____

    d) _____

DESIGNING FOR MEN
_____

78. As a professional, what type of styles should you recommend? _____

_____

79. Mustaches and beards can be a great way to _____ on male clients.

80. A man who is balding with closely trimmed hair could also look very good in a closely
    groomed _____

13 SHAMPOOING, RINSING, AND CONDITIONING

Date: _____

Rating: _____

Text Pages: 217-240

POINT TO PONDER:

> *"Formula For Success: Instruction + Example (X) Experience = Success"*
> *—unknown*

1. One of the most important experiences that a stylist provides is the _____ which can be heavenly, forgettable, or even a nightmare.

2. Shampooing is an important preliminary step that prepares the hair for a variety of services, it can also be

   a) _____

   b) _____

UNDERSTANDING SHAMPOO

3. The shampoo provides a good opportunity to _____ the client's hair and scalp.

4. What conditions should you check for during the shampoo?

   a) _____

   b) _____

   c) _____

   d) _____

   e) _____

   f) _____

   g) _____

   h) _____

5. The primary purpose of a shampoo is to _____ the hair and scalp prior to receiving a service.

6. To be effective, a shampoo must _____

_____ .

7. What will excessive shampooing do? _____

_____

8. Oily hair should be shampooed more often than normal or dry hair.

____ True

____ False

9. How should you select a shampoo for a client? _____

_____

10. Hair can usually be characterized as

a) _____

b) _____

c) _____

d) _____

11. Hair is not considered normal or virgin if it has been _____

_____

_____

12. A shampoo that is more _____ can have a pH ranging from 0 to 6.9.

13. A shampoo that is more _____ can have a pH rating of 7.1 or higher.

14. The _____ the pH rating, the stronger and harsher the shampoo.

15. A slightly _____ shampoo more closely matches the ideal pH of hair.

16. Water is classified as a _____ because it is capable of dissolving more substances than any other solvent known to science.

17. _____ is rain water or chemically softened water.

18. _____ is often in well water and contains certain minerals that lessen the ability of soap or shampoo to lather readily.

19. Water is the main ingredient in most shampoos.

____ True

____ False

20. Surfactant and detergent mean the same thing: _____

21. A surfactant molecule has two ends: a _____ or water-attracting "head," and a _____ or oil-attracting "tail."

22. During the shampoo process, the hydrophilic head attracts _____ and the lipophilic tail attracts _____

23. What does the process create? _____

_____

_____

24. Match the type of shampoo with its purpose for use:

____ 1. Acid-balanced shampoos   a) Contain special chemical or drugs to reduce dandruff

____ 2. Conditioning shampoos   b) Wash away excess oiliness, while keeping the hair from drying out

____ 3. Medicated shampoos   c) Designed to make the hair smooth and shiny

____ 4. Clarifying shampoos   d) Used to brighten, add slight color, eliminate unwanted tones

____ 5. Balancing shampoos   e) Special solutions available for hair enhancements

____ 6. Dry or powder shampoos   f) Balanced to the pH of skin and hair

____ 7. Color-enhancing shampoos   g) Cleanse the hair without the use of soap and water

____ 8. Shampoos for hairpieces/wigs   h) Cut through product buildup

25. _____ are special chemical agents applied to the hair to deposit protein or moisturizer, to help restore its strength and give it body, or to protect it against possible breakage.

26. Conditioners can heal damaged hair and can improve the quality of new hair growth.

____ True

____ False

27. Conditioners are also known as

a) _____

b) _____

28. What are the three basic types of conditioners?

    a) _____

    b) _____

    c) _____

29. What are humectants? _____

_____

30. Explain what conditioners do: _____

_____

31. _____ usually remain on the hair for a very short period of time and contain humectants to improve the appearance of dry, brittle hair.

32. Most conditioners have a pH range of _____ and restore the pH balance after an alkaline chemical treatment.

33. Heavier and creamier than instant conditioners, _____ have a longer application time of _____ .

34. _____ are designed to slightly increase hair diameter with a coating action, thereby _____ to the hair.

35. How do protein conditioners work? _____

_____

36. Protein conditioners

    a) _____

    b) _____

    c) _____

37. _____ , also known as hair masks or conditioning packs, are chemical mixtures of concentrated protein in a heavy base of moisturizer.

38. List and describe additional conditioning agents to be familiar with:

    a) _____

    b) _____

    c) _____

    d) _____

BRUSHING THE HAIR

39. Correct hair brushing

a) _____

b) _____

c) _____

40. When should hair brushing not be performed?

a) _____

b) _____

c) _____

41. What hair services should you not brush before?

a) _____

b) _____

c) _____

d) _____

14 | HAIRCUTTING

See Milady's Standard Cosmetology Practical Workbook

15 | HAIRSTYLING

See Milady's Standard Cosmetology Practical Workbook

16 | BRAIDING & BRAID EXTENSIONS

See Milady's Standard Cosmetology Practical Workbook

17 | WIGS & HAIR ENHANCEMENTS

See Milady's Standard Cosmetology Practical Workbook

18 CHEMICAL TEXTURE SERVICES

Date: _____

Rating: _____

Text Pages: 422-476

POINT TO PONDER:

"Don't confuse fame with success. Madonna is one; Helen Keller is the other."—Erma Bombeck

1. _____ services permanently alter the natural wave pattern of the hair.

2. Texture services can be used to add _____ to straight hair, _____ overly curly hair, or _____ coarse hair to make it more pliable and easier to work with.

3. Chemical textures services include

   a) _____

   b) _____

   c) _____

THE STRUCTURE OF HAIR

4. The _____ layer is the tough exterior layer of the hair. It surrounds the inner layers and _____ the hair from damage.

5. The cuticle is not directly involved in the texture or movement of the hair.

   ____ True

   ____ False

6. The _____ is the middle layer of the hair. It is responsible for the _____ and _____ of the human hair.

7. The _____ is often called the pith or core of the hair and does not play a role in structuring or restructuring the hair.

8. What does the term pH mean? _____

9. What does the pH scale measure? _____

10. What is the natural pH of hair? _____

11. Explain what chemical texturizers do to change the hair's natural curl pattern: _____

_____

_____

_____

12. Coarse, resistant hair with a strong, compact cuticle layer requires a highly alkaline chemical solution.

____ True

____ False

13. Match the following terms with its correct description:

____ 1. Amino acids   a) Formed by peptide bonds that are linked together

____ 2. Peptide bonds   b) Crosslinked polypeptide chains

____ 3. Polypeptide chains   c) Compounds made up of carbon, oxygen, hydrogen, and nitrogen

____ 4. Keratin   d) Weak physical side bonds that are the result of an attraction between opposite electrical charges

____ 5. Side bonds   e) Weak physical side bonds that are the result of an attraction between negative and positive electrical charges

____ 6. Disulfide bonds   f) Chemical side bonds that are formed when two sulfur type chains are joined together

____ 7. Salt bonds   g) Long, coiled polypeptide chains

____ 8. Hydrogen bonds   h) End bonds; link amino acids together in long chains

THE CLIENT CONSULTATION

14. Before proceeding with any service, you must first determine

a) _____

b) _____

15. To accurately communicate with your client you must

a) _____

_____

b) _____

c) _____

d) _____

e) _____

_____

f) _____

g) _____

_____

h) _____

_____

16. Metallic salts are not compatible with permanent waving.

____ True

____ False

17. Metallic salts leave a coating on the hair that may

a) _____

b) _____

c) _____

18. Explain the procedure to determine if there are metallic salts present on the hair:

_____

_____

_____

_____

_____

19. Client records should include a complete evaluation of

a) _____

b) _____

c) _____

d) _____

20. If client release forms do not release the school or salon from all responsibility for any damages that may occur, what is the purpose? _____

_____

_____

21. When performing an analysis of the scalp, what should you look for? _____

_____

22. It is okay to proceed with chemical texture services if there are minor skin abrasions or scalp disease.

____ True

____ False

23. The five most important factors to consider in a hair analysis are

a) _____

b) _____

c) _____

d) _____

e) _____

24. Match the following term with its correct description:

____ 1. Texture   a) The hair's ability to absorb moisture

____ 2. Density   b) The diameter of a hair strand

____ 3. Porosity   c) How the hair naturally lays

____ 4. Elasticity   d) The thickness or number of hairs per square inch

____ 5. Growth direction   e) How far the hair stretches before breaking and how well it returns to its original shape

25. Match the following hair textures with the phrase that best describes it:

____ 1. coarse hair   a) More fragile; easier to process

____ 2. medium hair   b) Most common hair texture; does not pose any problems or concerns

____ 3. fine hair   c) Usually more resistant to processing

26. _____ measures the number of hairs per square inch on the head to determine whether a client has _____ _____ , or _____ hair.

27. Coarse hair naturally looks _____ and _____.

28. The degree of porosity is directly related to the condition of the _____ layer.

29. Match the following degree of porosity with its description:

____ 1. resistant hair   a) Has a raised cuticle layer that easily absorbs

____ 2. normal porosity   b) Has a tight, compact cuticle that resist penetration

____ 3. overly porous   c) Neither resistant nor overly porous

30. _____ is an indication of the strength of the side bonds that hold the individual fibers of the hair in place.

31. More than any other single factor, the elasticity of the hair determines its ability to

_____.

32. How is elasticity usually classified? _____

33. Wet hair with normal elasticity can stretch up to what percentage of its original length, then return to the same length without breaking?

____ a) 10%

____ b) 25%

____ c) 50%

____ d) 75%

34. The individual growth direction of the hair causes _____ that influence the finished hairstyle and must be considered when selecting the base direction and wrapping pattern for each permanent wave.

PERMANENT WAVING

35. What are the two steps of the permanent wave process?

a) _____

b) _____

_____

36. In permanent waving, the size of the rod determines the _____.

37. _____ are the most common type of perm rod. They have a smaller _____ in the center that increases to a larger circumference on the ends.

38. Concave rods produce a _____ in the center and a _____ on either side of the strand.

39. _____ are equal in diameter along their entire length or curling area.

40. Straight rods produce a _____ along the entire width of the strand.

41. _____ are usually about 12″ long with a uniform diameter along the entire length.

42. What allows these soft foam roads to bend into almost any shape? _____

_____

43. The _____ or _____ rod is usually about 12″ long with a uniform diameter along the entire length of the rod.

44. _____ are absorbent papers used to control the ends of the hair when wrapping and winding hair on the perm rods.

45. Why is important to extend end papers beyond the ends of the hair? _____

_____

46. List the most common end paper techniques and explain each:

a) _____

_____

b) _____

_____

c) _____

47. All perm wraps begin by sectioning the hair into _____

48. How do you determine the size, shape, and direction of these panels? _____

_____

49. Each panel is divided into subsections called _____ .

50. _____ refers to the position of the rod in relation to its base section, and it is determined by the angle at which the hair is wrapped.

51. Rods can be wrapped

a) _____

b) _____

c) _____

52. For on base placement, the hair is wrapped _____ beyond perpendicular to its base section.

53. Half off base placement refers to wrapping the hair at a _____ angle or straight out from the center of the section.

54. Half off base placement _____ stress and tension on the hair.

55. Off base placement refers to wrapping the hair at _____ below the center of the base section.

56. Which placement creates the least amount of volume and results in curl patterns that begin farthest away from the scalp? _____

57. Base direction refers to the angle at which the rod is positioned on the head:

_____

58. Why is it important to remember to wrap in the natural direction of hair growth?

_____

59. The two methods of wrapping the hair around the perm rod are

a) _____

b) _____

60. In which method is the hair strand wound around the rod, going from the ends to the scalp? _____

61. Which method produces a uniform curl from the scalp to ends? _____

62. What is a double tool or piggyback wrap, and when is it beneficial? _____

_____

_____

63. What is the benefit for wrapping long hair in a piggyback wrap? _____

_____

64. What does an alkaline permanent waving solution do? _____

_____

65. Once the solution is in the cortex, what occurs? _____

_____

66. What is a reduction reaction? _____

_____

67. What is a reduction reaction in permanent waving? _____

68. Explain the chemical process of re-forming hair:

a) _____

b) _____
_____

c) _____
_____

d) _____
_____

69. What is the reducing agent used in permanent waving solutions? _____

70. _____ is the most common reducing agent.

71. The strength of the permanent waving solution is determined by _____
_____

72. Why is ammonia added to the thioglycolic acid product? _____
_____
_____

73. The new chemical created is called _____ and is the active
ingredient or reducing agent in alkaline permanents.

74. The first _____ were developed in 1941 and relied on the same ATG that is
still used today.

75. Most alkaline waves have a pH between (_____

76. _____ is an acid with a low pH and is the primary reducing
agent in all modern acid waves.

77. The first _____ were introduced in the early 1970s and have a pH between
_____ . They require _____ to speed up processing.

78. The three separate components of all acid waves are

a) _____

b) _____

c) _____

79. Most acid waves today have a pH between

___ a) 5.8 and 6.2

___ b) 6.8 and 7.2

___ c) 7.8 and 8.2

___ d) 8.8 and 9.2

80. _____ process more quickly and produce firmer curls than true acid waves.

81. _____ create an exothermic chemical reaction that heats up the solution and speeds up the processing.

82. Exothermic waves have three components:

a) _____

b) _____

c) _____

83. Mixing an oxidizer with the permanent waving solution causes _____

_____

84. _____ are activated by an outside heat source, usually a conventional hood type dryer.

85. _____ use an ingredient that does not evaporate as readily as ammonia, so there is very little odor associated with their use.

86. _____ use an ingredient other than ATG as the primary reducing agent.

87. The use of sulfates, sulfites, and bisulfites present an alternative to ATG known as

_____.

88. The strength of any permanent wave is based on the concentration of its _____

_____.

89. The amount of processing during a permanent wave is determined by the _____ of the permanent waving solution.

90. In permanent waving, most of the processing takes place as soon as the solution _____ within the first 5 to 10 minutes.

91. What does the additional processing time allow? _____

_____

92. When does over processing usually occur? _____

93. Resistant hair may not become completely saturated with just one application of waving solution.

____ True

____ False

94. What occurs if the hair is under processed? _____

_____

95. _____ is the process of stopping the action of a permanent waving solution and rebuilds the hair into its new form.

96. The two important functions of neutralization are

a) _____

b) _____

97. The most common neutralizer is _____

98. When rinsing the perm solution from the hair, how long should you rinse? _____

_____

99. If the hair is insufficiently blotted, what will occur? _____

_____

100. Oxidative reactions can _____ hair color, especially at an alkaline pH.

101. When rinsing the hair, you should always use hot water.

____ True

____ False

102. When rinsing the hair, use a gentle stream of water.

____ True

____ False

103. How should you towel blot the hair after rinsing? _____

104. Always adjust any rods that have become _____ prior to applying the neutralizer.

105. _____ breaks disulfide bonds by adding hydrogen atoms to the sulfur atoms. _____ rebuilds the disulfide bonds by removing the extra hydrogen atoms.

106. List the safety precautions for permanent waving.

a) _____

b) _____

   _____

c) _____

d) _____

e) _____

f) _____

g) _____

h) _____

i) _____

j) _____

k) _____

l) _____

CHEMICAL HAIR RELAXERS

107. _____ is the process of rearranging the basic structure of extremely curly hair into a straighter or smoother form.

108. The chemistry of thio relaxers and permanent waving is exactly the same.

____ True

____ False

109. The two most common types of hair relaxers are _____ and

   _____ .

110. Extremely curly hair grows in long twisted spirals or coils, with the thinnest and weakest sections of the hair strands located at their twists.

____ True

____ False

111. _____ usually have a pH above 10 and a higher concentrate of ammonium thioglycolate than is used in permanent waving.

112. The _____ used with thio relaxers is an oxidizing agent, usually hydrogen peroxide, just as in permanents.

113. The _____ is the active ingredient in all hydroxide relaxers.

114. All hydroxide relaxers are very strong alkalis that can swell the hair up to twice its normal diameter.

___ True

___ False

115. Why are hydroxide relaxers not compatible with thio relaxers? _____

_____

116. Hydroxide relaxers remove one atom of sulfur from a disulfide bond, converting it into a lanthionine body by a process called _____

117. The neutralization of hydroxide relaxers involves oxidation.

___ True

___ False

118. What does the application of an acid-balanced shampoo or normalizing lotion do?

_____

119. _____ are ionic compounds formed by a metal—sodium (Na), potassium (K), or lithium (Li)—which is combined with oxygen (O) and hydrogen (H).

120. Sodium hydroxide relaxers are commonly called _____.

121. _____ and _____ relaxers are often advertised and sold as "no mix–no lye" relaxers.

122. _____ relaxers are usually advertised and sold as "no lye" relaxers.

123. Guanidine hydroxide relaxers straighten the hair completely, with much less scalp irritation than other hydroxide relaxers.

___ True

___ False

124. _____ and _____ are sometimes used as low-pH hair relaxers.

125. _____ is an oily cream used to protect the skin and scalp during hair relaxing.

126. _____ require the application of base cream to the entire scalp prior to the application of the relaxer.

127. _____ do not require application of a protective base. They contain a base cream that is designed to melt at body temperature.

128. List the different strengths of relaxers and what each is formulated for:

a) _____

b) _____

c) _____

19 HAIRCOLORING

Date: _____

Rating: _____

Text Pages: 477-528

POINT TO PONDER:

"The difference between a successful person and others is not a lack of strength, not a lack of knowledge, but rather a lack of will."
—*Vince Lombardi*

1. One of the most creative, challenging and popular salon services is _____ .

2. Haircolor is both a _____ and an _____ .

3. A skilled haircolorist needs to become an expert in the following processes:

   a) _____

   b) _____

   c) _____

   d) _____

   e) _____

   f) _____

4. Statistics show that clients who have haircuts stay with their stylist for an average of
   _____ ,   while clients who receive color services stay with their stylist for _____ .

WHY PEOPLE COLOR THEIR HAIR

5. What are a few reasons clients color their hair?

   a) _____

   b) _____

   c) _____

   d) _____
   _____

   e) _____

HAIR FACTS

6. What is the determining factor in choosing which haircolor to use, that will affect the quality and ultimate success of the service? _____

7. Name and describe the three main parts of the hair:

   a) _____

   _____

   b) _____

   _____

   c) _____

8. Which part of the hair contains the natural pigment? _____

9. Hair _____ is determined by the diameter of the individual hair strand.

10. In fine hair the melanin granules are grouped more _____ so hair takes color _____ and can look darker.

11. Which hair type can take longer to process? _____

12. Hair _____ is the number of hairs per square inch, ranging from thin to thick.

13. _____ is the ability of the hair to absorb moisture.

14. Match the following degrees of porosity with its description:

    ____ 1. Low porosity   a) The cuticle is lifted; hair takes color quickly

    ____ 2. Average porosity   b) The cuticle is tight; hair is resistant

    ____ 3. High porosity   c) The cuticle is slightly raised; hair is normal and processes in average amount of time

IDENTIFYING NATURAL HAIR COLOR AND TONE

15. What is the most important step in becoming a good colorist? _____

    _____

16. The two main types of melanin in the cortex are

    a) _____

    b) _____

17. Natural hair color can be a combination of both types of melanin.

    ____ True

    ____ False

18. _____ is the pigment that lies under the natural hair color and must be taken into consideration when you select a haircolor.

19. _____ is the unit of measurement used to identify the lightness or darkness of a color.

20. Haircolor levels are arranged on a scale of 1 to 10, with 1 being the _____ and 10 being the _____ .

21. _____ , or the hue of color, refers to the balance of the color and can be described as _____ , or _____ .

22. _____ tones reflect light so they look lighter than the level they are. These tones are

    a) _____

    b) _____

    c) _____

    d) _____

23. _____ tones are colors that absorb more light, so they look deeper than their actual level. These tones are

    a) _____

    b) _____

    c) _____

24. _____ tones are a cross between cool and warm tones. They are described as _____ or _____ .

25. A color can be as bright or as soft as desired; color _____ serve this purpose.

26. Gray hair is limited to the aging process.

    ___ True
    ___ False

27. Gray hair requires special attention in formulating haircolor.

    ___ True
    ___ False

28. What are all colors developed from? _____

29. A _____ is the predominant tone of a color.

30. Haircolor with a violet base color will deliver _____ and minimize _____.

31. Haircolor with a red-orange base will create _____.

32. The _____ is a system for understanding color.

33. The Law of Color states that when combing colors, you will always get the same result from the same combination.

    ____ True

    ____ False

34. _____ are pure colors that cannot be achieved from a mixture.

35. The primary colors are _____

36. _____ colors are created from the three primary colors.

    a) Some

    b) All

    c) Most

    d) A few

37. Colors with a pure dominance of blue are _____ colors, and colors with a predominance of red are _____ colors.

38. _____ is the strongest of the primary colors and is the only _____ primary color.

39. _____ is the medium primary color.

40. Red added to blue-based colors will cause them to appear _____.

    a) Darker

    b) Lighter

    c) Trendier

    d) Classic

41. Red added to yellow colors will cause them to become _____.

    a) Darker

    b) Lighter

    c) Trendier

    d) Classic

42. The weakest of the primary colors is _____.

43. When you add yellow to other colors, the resulting color will look _____.

    a) Deeper and darker

    b) Lighter and brighter

    c) More youthful

    d) More sophisticated

44. When all three colors are present in equal proportions, the resulting color is black, white, or gray, depending on _____

45. A _____ color is a color obtained by mixing equal parts of two primary colors.

46. The secondary colors are _____

47. Green is an equal combination of _____

48. Orange is an equal combination of _____

49. Violet is an equal combination of _____

50. A _____ is an intermediate color achieved by mixing a secondary color and its neighboring primary color on the color wheel in _____ parts.

51. Tertiary colors include

    a) _____

    b) _____

    c) _____

    d) _____

    e) _____

    f) _____

52. Natural looking haircolor is made up of a combination of _____ colors.

53. _____ are a primary and secondary color positioned directly opposite each other on the color wheel.

54. Next to each color below, list its complementary color:

Blue   _____

Red   _____

Yellow   _____

55. Complementary colors _____ each other.

56. Place a "P," "S," and "T" on the color wheel in their proper places to signify primary, secondary and tertiary colors.

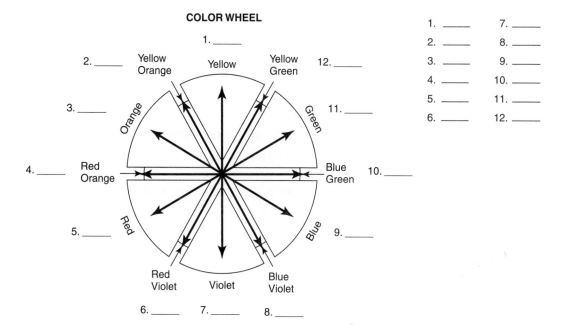

COLOR WHEEL

1. _____

2. _____   Yellow Orange   Yellow   Yellow Green   12. _____

3. _____   Orange

4. _____   Red Orange   Blue Green   10. _____

5. _____   Red   Blue   9. _____

Red Violet   Violet   Blue Violet

6. _____   7. _____   8. _____

11. _____

Green

1. _____   7. _____
2. _____   8. _____
3. _____   9. _____
4. _____   10. _____
5. _____   11. _____
6. _____   12. _____

TYPES OF HAIRCOLOR

57. Name the two categories haircoloring products generally fall into: _____

_____

58. The oxidative category has two classifications: _____ ; the nonoxidative category has two classifications: _____ .

59. How long before a color service should a patch test be given? _____

   a) 12 to 24 minutes

   b) 24 to 48 minutes

   c) 12 to 24 hours

   d) 24 to 48 hours

60. Hair lightening, also referred to as _____ or _____ , is the chemical process involving the diffusion of the natural hair color pigment or artificial color from the hair.

61. All permanent haircolor products and lighteners contain both a _____ or _____ and an _____.

62. The role of the alkalizing ingredient is to

a) _____

b) _____

c) _____

63. When the haircolor containing the alkalizing ingredient is combined with the developer, the peroxide becomes alkaline and decomposes or breaks up; lightening occurs when the alkaline peroxide breaks up the _____.

64. Temporary haircolor is a good choice for those who wish to _____ yellow hair or unwanted tones.

65. The pigments in _____ are large and do not penetrate the cuticle layer, allowing only a coating action that may be removed by _____.

66. Temporary haircolors are nonoxidation colors that make only a physical change, not a chemical change, in the hair shaft.

____ True

____ False

67. List the products that provide temporary hair color:

a) _____

b) _____

c) _____

d) _____

e) _____

_____

68. _____ is formulated to last through several shampoos, depending on the hair's porosity.

69. How does semi-permanent haircolor work? _____

_____

_____

70. Semi-permanent haircolor is required to be mixed with a peroxide.

    ____ True

    ____ False

71. Demipermanent haircolor is also called _____ . It is formulated to _____ , but not lift color and is often called a non-lift–deposit-only color.

72. No-lift deposition only haircolors are ideal for

    a) _____

    b) _____

    c) _____

    d) _____

73. No-lift–deposit-only haircolor is available as a _____ .

74. _____ can lighten and deposit color at the same time and in one process and are usually mixed with a higher volume developer.

75. Permanent hair color products generally contain uncolored dye precursors, also known as _____ .

76. Dye precursors are small and can _____ into the hair shaft.

77. Molecules are trapped within the _____ of the hair and cannot be shampooed out.

78. Permanent hair coloring products are regarded as the best products for covering _____ hair.

79. Permanent hair coloring simultaneously removes _____ from the hair through the action of lightening while adding _____ to both the gray and the pigmented hair.

80. Natural or _____ are natural colors obtained from the leaves or bark of plants. An example of this type of color is _____ .

81. Do natural colors lighten the hair? _____

82. If a client who has used natural haircolor comes into the salon, can you apply additional chemical products over the top of natural haircolors? _____

83. _____ , also called gradual colors, contain metal salts and change hair color gradually by progressive build-up and exposure to hair, creating a dull metallic appearance.

84. Historically, who have metallic haircolors been marketed to? _____

85. A _____ is an oxidizing agent that, when mixed with an oxidative hair color, supplies the necessary oxygen gas to develop color molecules and create a change in hair color.

86. Developers are also called _____.

87. The pH of developer is _____

    a) between 1.0 and 2.3

    b) between 2.5 and 4.5

    c) between 6.5 and 7.5

    d) between 8.5 and 9.5

88. Name the most commonly used developer on the market. _____

89. _____ measures the concentration and strength of hydrogen peroxide.

90. The lower the volume, the _____; the higher the volume, the _____ _____.

91. Describe the common use of the following volumes of hydrogen peroxide:

    a) 20 volume   _____

    b) 30 volume   _____

    c) 40 volume   _____
                        _____

92. _____ lighten hair by dispersing, dissolving, and decolorizing the natural hair pigment.

93. What happens when hydrogen peroxide is mixed into the lightener formula? _____ _____ . The process is known as _____.

94. Hair lighteners are used to

    a) _____

    b) _____

    c) _____

    d) _____

    e) _____

95. How many stages of color may hair go through as it lightens? _____

    a) Three

    b) Five

    c) Eight

    d) Ten

96. Why would a colorist choose to decolorize a client's hair before tinting?_____

_____

_____

97. _____ are traditional semi-permanent, demi-permanent, and permanent hair color products that are used primarily on prelighted hair to achieve pale and delicate colors after the _____ process.

98. All hair will go through all 10 degrees of decolorization.

    ____ True

    ____ False

99. How can you tell if you have damaged the hair during the decolorization process?

_____

CONSULTATION

100. A haircolor _____ is the most critical part of the color service.

101. During the consultation, your client will communicate _____.
It is important that you _____ so you can make an appropriate recommendation.

102. What is the single most reliable way to ensure a client's satisfaction? _____

_____

103. Wall color should be _____ or _____ when performing the color consultation.

104. What is the purpose of the client information card? _____

_____

105. List some of the questions you might ask the client during the consultation:

    a) _____

    b) _____

    c) _____

106. A _____ is used by many salons when providing chemical services. Its purpose is to explain to clients that if their hair is in questionable condition, it may not withstand the requested chemical treatment.

SELECTING HAIRCOLOR

107. List the four basic questions you should ask when formulating a haircolor:

   a) _____

   b) _____

   c) _____

   d) _____

108. List the two methods used for the application of permanent haircolor:

   a) _____

   b) _____

109. When using the brush and bowl technique, the bowl should be a _____ mixing bowl.

110. When working with hair color, you will have to determine whether your clients have any allergies or sensitivities to the mixture. To do this you will administer a _____ also known as a _____ .

111. How many hours prior to application of aniline haircolor should a patch test be given?

   _____

   a) 5 to 10

   b) 12 to 18

   c) 24 to 48

   d) 62 to 78

112. The color used for the patch test must be _____

   _____

113. A negative skin test result will show _____

114. A positive skin test result will show _____

HAIRCOLOR APPLICATION

115. A clearly defined system makes for the _____ and for the safest and most satisfactory results.

116. A _____ will tell you how the hair will react to the formula and how long the formula should be left on the hair.

117. When is the strand test performed? _____

118. There is only one correct method for applying temporary haircolor.

___ True

___ False

119. Semipermanent colors do not contain the_____ necessary to lift. So they only

_____

120. When applying semipermanent over existing color, remember that it always

_____.

121. How is the application procedure for demipermanent haircolor determined?_____

_____

122. Why does gray hair present a challenge when formulating no lift deposit only haircolor?

_____

_____

123. Permanent hair color applications are classified as either _____-process or _____-process.

124. _____ is a process that lightens and deposits color in a single application.

125. The first time the hair is colored is referred to as a _____

126. A single-process tint that usually contains a nonammonia color and adds shine and tone to the hair is a _____

127. As the hair grows, you will need to _____ to keep it looking attractive and to avoid a two-toned effect.

128. In a retouch, the tint should be applied to _____

   a) The hair at the ends only

   b) The hair at the mid-shaft

   c) Only the new growth only

   d) The prelightened hair only

129. A visible line separating colored hair from new growth is called _____

   a) Hyperpigmentation

   b) Hypopigmentation

   c) Line of demarcation

   d) Line of decolorization

130. If the client asks for a dramatically lighter color, what has to be done? _____

_____

131. _____ , also known as two-step coloring, is a technique requiring two separate procedures in which the hair is prelightened and then toned.

132. Why is a wider range of haircolor possible during a double-process high lift coloring?

_____

LIGHTENING TECHNIQUES

133. What are the three forms of lightener? _____

134. Oil and cream are _____ , which can be used directly on the scalp.

135. Powder lighteners are _____ , which cannot be used on the scalp.

136. Why are oil and cream lighteners the most popular? _____

137. Which lightener is the mildest? _____

138. List the features of cream lighteners:

   a) _____

   b) _____

   c) _____

139. _____ contain a powdered oxidizer and/or the same persulfate salts that are used in powdered off the scalp hair lighteners.

140 _____ lighteners are strong enough for high lift blonding, but gentle enough to be used on the scalp.

141. What does an activator do? _____

_____

142. How many activators can be used for on-the-scalp lightener applications? _____

143. _____ are strong, fast-acting lighteners in powdered form.

144. Why should most powdered lighteners not be used for retouch services? _____

_____

145. Name the factors that affect processing time for lighteners:

a) _____

_____

b) _____

c) _____

_____

d) _____

e) _____

146. To determine the processing time for your lightening service, the condition of the hair after lightening, and the end results, you should perform a _____.

147. What is new growth? _____

_____

148. What will occur if lighteners are overlapped during a retouch? _____

_____

USING TONERS

149. Toners are used primarily on prelightened hair to achieve _____ colors.

150. What is most often used as a toner? _____

151. The _____ pigment is the color that remains in the hair after lightening.

152. As a general rule, the paler the color you are seeking, _____

_____.

153. Why should you not prelighten past the pale yellow stage? _____

_____

SPECIAL EFFECTS HAIR COLORING

154. Special effects hair coloring refers to any technique that involves _____ _____.

155. Coloring some of the hair strands lighter than the natural color to add the illusion of depth is called _____.

156. Coloring strands of hair darker than the natural color is called _____ _____.

157. Name the three most frequently used techniques for achieving highlights:

   a) _____

   b) _____

   c) _____

158. The _____ involves pulling clean strands of hair through a perforated cap with a thin plastic or metal hook.

159. The _____ of strands pulled through determines the degree of highlighting or lowlighting you can achieve.

160. The _____ involves coloring selected strands of hair by slicing or weaving out sections, placing them on foil or plastic wrap, applying lightener or color, and sealing them in the foil or plastic wrap.

161. _____ involves taking a narrow, ⅛″ section of hair by making a straight part at the scalp, positioning the hair over the foil, and applying lightener or color.

162. In _____ , selected strands are picked up from a narrow section of hair with a zigzag motion of the comb, and lightener or color is applied only to these strands.

163. The _____ or the _____ technique involves the painting of a lightener directly onto clean, styled hair.

164. To avoid affecting untreated hair, you may choose

   a) _____
   _____

   b) _____

   c) _____

165. _____ are prepared by combining permanent haircolor, hydrogen peroxide, and shampoo.

166. When should you use a highlighting shampoo? _____

_____

SPECIAL CHALLENGES IN HAIR COLOR/CORRECTIVE COLORING

167. A skilled colorist will occasionally have a problem in haircolor that can't be predicted. This may be due to _____ .

168. What can cause gray hair to have a yellow cast?

a) _____

b) _____

c) _____

d) _____

169. Which of the following should not be used to correct a yellow discoloration?

_____

a) Lightener

b) Tint remover

c) Violet-based colors

d) Orange-based colors

170. Will hair color at a level 8 or lighter give complete gray coverage? Why or why not?

_____

_____

171. What considerations should be taken into account when formulating haircolor for gray hair?

a) _____

b) _____

c) _____

172. List the tips when working with gray hair:

a) _____

b) _____

c) _____

d) _____

173. _____ raises the cuticle layer of gray or resistant hair to allow for better penetration of color. It is considered a _____ haircoloring service.

174. List the rules for effective color application:

a) _____

b) _____

c) _____

d) _____

e) _____

f) _____

g) _____

175. What are the characteristics of damaged hair?

a) _____

b) _____

c) _____

d) _____

e) _____

f) _____

g) _____

176. When dealing with damaged hair, what should occur before proceeding with the chemical service? _____

177. When dealing with damaged hair

a) _____

b) _____

c) _____

d) _____

e) _____

178. _____ help equalize porosity.

179. The two main types of fillers are

    a) _____

    b) _____

180. _____ fillers are used to recondition damaged, overly porous hair and equalize porosity.

181. _____ equalize porosity and deposit color in one application.

HAIRCOLORING SAFETY PRECAUTION

182. List the haircoloring safety precautions:

    a) _____

    b) _____

    c) _____

    d) _____

    e) _____

    f) _____

    g) _____

    h) _____

    i) _____

    j) _____

    k) _____

    l) _____

    m) _____

    n) _____

20 SKIN DISEASES & DISORDERS

Date: _____

Rating: _____

Text Pages: 529-545

POINT TO PONDER:

"Excellence is not an act, it is a habit."—***Aristotle***

AGING OF THE SKIN

1. Name the factors that influence the aging of the skin:

    a) _____

    b) _____

    c) _____

    d) _____

2. What percentage of aging is determined by heredity?

    ____ a) 15%

    ____ b) 25%

    ____ c) 40%

    ____ d) 50%

3. Approximately 80% to 85% of our aging is caused by the _____

4. As we age, the _____ and _____ of the skin naturally weaken.

5. The ultraviolet rays of the sun reach the skin in two different forms, _____ and _____ rays.

6. UVA rays, also called _____ , are deep penetrating rays that weaken the collagen and elastin fibers, causing _____ in the tissues.

7. UVB rays, also referred to as the _____ , cause sunburns and tanning by affecting the melanocytes.

8. What helps protect the skin from the sun's ultraviolet rays? _____

9. List the precautions to take when exposed to the sun:

a) _____

b) _____

c) _____

d) _____

e) _____

f) _____

g) _____

   _____

h) _____

10. In addition to the sun, what else plays a role in how the skin ages? _____

    _____

11. What is the best defense against pollutants? _____

    _____

    _____

12. What affect does each of the following have on the skin?

    Smoking   _____

    Nicotine   _____

                    _____

                    _____

                    _____

                    _____

13. Over time, capillaries dilate, called _____ and weakening of the fragile
    capillary walls will cause them to become distended.

14. Damage done by lifestyle changes is hard to reverse or diminish.

    ____ True

    ____ False

DISORDERS OF THE SKIN

15. A _____ is a mark on the skin that could indicate an injury or damage that changes
    the structure of tissues or organs.

16. The three types of lesions are

    a) _____

    b) _____

    c) _____

17. Which two are the cosmetologists concerned with? _____

18. Match each of the following primary lesions with its description:

    ___ 1. Bulla   a) A spot or discoloration on the skin

    ___ 2. Cyst   b) A small blister or sac containing clear fluid; just beneath the
                              epidermis

    ___ 3. Macule   c) A swelling

    ___ 4. Papule   d) A large blister containing a watery fluid

    ___ 5. Pustule   e) An itchy, swollen lesion lasting only a few hours

    ___ 6. Tubercle   f) An inflamed pimple containing pus

    ___ 7. Tumor   g) A closed, abnormally developed sac, containing fluid, pus,
                              or semifluid

    ___ 8. Vesicle   h) A small, circumscribed elevation on the skin containing no fluid

    ___ 9. Wheel   i) An abnormal rounded, solid lump, within or under the skin

19. A _____ lesion is one that develops in the later stages of disease.

20. Identify the secondary skin lesions as illustrated:

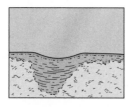 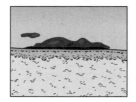

_____   _____

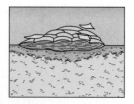 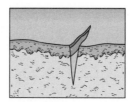 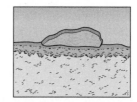

_____   _____   _____

21. Match each of the following secondary lesions with its description:

___ 1. Crust   a) A skin sore or abrasion produced by scratching or scraping

___ 2. Excoriation   b) A thick scar resulting from excessive growth of fibrous tissue

___ 3. Fissure   c) Light-colored, slightly raised mark on the skin formed after injury

___ 4. Keloid   d) An open lesion on the skin or mucous membrane of the body

___ 5. Scale   e) Any thin plate of epidermal flakes, dry or oily

___ 6. Scar   f) A crack in the skin that penetrates the dermis

___ 7. Ulcer   g) Dead cells that form over a wound or blemish while it is healing

22. Match each of the following disorders of the sebaceous glands with its description:

___ 1. Comedo   a) A skin condition caused by inflammation of the sebaceous glands

___ 2. Milia   b) A chronic condition appearing primarily on the cheeks and nose

___ 3. Acne   c) A hair follicle filled with keratin and sebum

___ 4. Seborrheic dermatitis   d) Chronic inflammation of the sebaceous glands

___ 5. Asteatosis   e) A sebaceous cyst or fatty tumor

___ 6. Rosacea   f) Benign, keratin-filled cysts

___ 7. Steatoma   g) A condition of dry, scaly skin due to a deficiency of sebum

23. Match each of following disorders of the sudoriferous glands with its description:

___ 1. Anhidrosis   a) Foul-smelling perspiration

___ 2. Bromhidrosis   b) Excessive sweating

___ 3. Hyperhidrosis   c) Deficiency in perspiration

___ 4. Miliaria rubra   d) Prickly heat; acute inflammatory disorder of the sweat glands

24. Match each of the following skin condition with its description:

___ 1. Dermatitis   a) Fever blister or cold sore

___ 2. Eczema   b) Inflammatory condition of the skin

___ 3. Herpes simplex   c) Characterized by red patches, covered with silver white scales

___ 4. Psoriasis   d) Inflammatory, painful itching disease

25. Match each of the following skin pigmentation with its description:

___ 1. Albinism   a) Increased pigmentation on the skin

___ 2. Chloasm   b) Small or large malformation of the skin due to abnormal pigmentation

___ 3. Lentigines   c) Absence of melanin pigment of the body

___ 4. Leukoderma   d) Abnormal brown or wine-colored skin discoloration

___ 5. Nevus   e) Change in pigmentation caused by exposure to the sun or ultraviolet rays

___ 6. Stain   f) Milky white spots of skin

___ 7. Tan   g) Skin disorder characterized by light abnormal patches

___ 8. Vitiligo   h) Technical term for freckles

26. _____ of the skin is an abnormal growth of the skin.

27. Match the following with its description:

___ 1. Keratoma   a) A small, brownish spot or blemish

___ 2. Mole   b) Technical term for wart

___ 3. Skin tag   c) Small brown or flesh-colored outgrowth of the skin

___ 4. Verruca   d) An acquired, superficial, thickened patch of epidermis

28. _____ is the most common type of skin cancer and is the least severe.

29. _____ is more serious and often is characterized by scaly red papules or nodules.

30. _____ is the most serious form of skin cancer and is often characterized by black or dark brown patches and may appear uneven in texture, jagged, or raised.

AVOIDING SKIN PROBLEMS

31. _____ is the medical term for abnormal skin inflammation. The most common skin disease for cosmetologists is _____ .

32. If the skin is irritated by a substance, it is called _____ contact dermatitis. If one develops an allergy to a product, it is called _____ contact dermatitis.

33. Prolonged, repeated, or long-term exposure can cause anyone to become sensitive, usually caused by _____ .

34. What are the most likely places allergies may occur?

    a) _____

    b) _____

    c) _____

35. _____ is a greatly increased or exaggerated sensitivity to products.

36. Explain what occurs when the skin is damaged by irritating substances: _____

    _____

    _____

37. What is a very common salon irritant? _____ Why? _____

    _____ How can it be

    avoided? _____

    _____

21 HAIR REMOVAL

See Milady's Standard Cosmetology Practical Workbook

22 FACIALS

Date: _____

Rating: _____

Text Pages: 561-602

POINT TO PONDER:

*"Change is inevitable. Growth is optional."—**unknown***

1. Facial treatments can be very relaxing and offer many improvements to the _____ of the skin.

2. Proper skin care can make oily skin look _____ ; dry skin look and feel more _____ ; and aging skin look _____

SKIN ANALYSIS AND CONSULTATION

3. _____ is a very important part of the facial treatment because it determines what type of the skin the client has, the condition of the skin, and what type of treatment the client's skin needs.

4. The opportunity to ask the client questions about his or her health and skin care history and to advise the client about appropriate home care products and treatments is during the _____ .

5. Before beginning the analysis, what must the client fill out? _____

_____

6. A _____ is a condition the client has or a treatment the client is undergoing that might cause a negative side effect during the facial treatment.

7. List the main contraindications to look for:

a) _____

_____

b) _____

c) _____

d) _____

e) _____

f) _____

g) _____

h) _____

i) _____

j) _____

8. What additional information can you obtain when the client completes the health-screening form?

a) _____

b) _____

c) _____

d) _____

e) _____

_____

f) _____

9. Why should health-screening forms be kept separately and secured? _____

_____

SKIN CARE PRODUCTS

10. _____ are designed to clean the surface of the skin and to remove makeup.

11. List and describe the two types of cleansers:

a) _____

_____

b) _____

_____

12. Foaming cleansers contain surfactants, also known as _____ , that cause the product to foam and rinse easily.

13. Toners, also known as _____ or _____ , are designed to lower the pH of the skin after cleansing and to help remove excess cleansing milk.

14. Toners may contain ingredients that help to

    a) _____

    b) _____

15. Fresheners and astringents are usually stronger products with higher _____ content and are used to treat _____

16. How are toning products applied? _____

17. Describe what exfoliants do _____

18. What are exfoliants used for? _____

    _____

    _____

19. Cosmetologists are allowed to use products that remove dead surface cells from the _____ . Deeper, surgical level peels can only be administered by

    _____ .

20. List the two basic types of exfoliants:

    a) _____

    b) _____

21. Mechanical exfoliants work by physically bumping off _____ build-up.

22. List some examples of mechanical exfoliants:

    a) _____

    b) _____

    c) _____

    d) _____

23. How do chemical exfoliants work? _____

24. List two popular exfoliating chemicals:

    a) _____

    b) _____

25. Describe how these acids work: _____

_____

_____

_____

_____

26. Salon alphahydroxy acid exfoliants are often referred to as _____ .

27. _____ are another type of chemical exfoliant. They are known as _____
_____ or protein-dissolving agents.

28. How do enzyme peels work? _____

29. Enzyme products are made from plant-extracted enzymes from

a) _____

b) _____

c) _____

d) _____

30. What are the two basic types of keratolytic enzyme peels? _____

31. Proper exfoliation may improve the appearance of

a) _____

b) _____

c) _____

d) _____

e) _____

f) _____

g) _____

32. _____ are products that help increase the moisture content of the skin surface.

33. Moisturizers are mixtures of _____ , also known as hydrators, which are oily or fatty ingredients that block moisture from leaving the skin.

34. Moisturizers that are most often in lotion form and contain smaller amounts of emollient are for _____

35. Moisturizers that are often in the form of a heavier cream and contain more emollients are for _____

36. What is the most important habit to benefit the skin? _____

_____

37. An _____ or higher is considered to be a thorough sunscreen strength.

38. Night treatment products are usually more _____ products designed to be used at night to treat _____.

39. _____ and _____ are concentrated products that generally contain higher amounts of ingredients that have an effect on the skin appearance.

40. Lubricants to make the skin slippery during massage are called _____.

41. _____ are products that are applied to the skin for a short time but have more immediate effects.

42. Match the following types of mask with its intended use:

____ 1. Clay-based masks

____ 2. Cream masks

____ 3. Gel masks

____ 4. Alginate masks

____ 5. Paraffin wax masks

____ 6. Modelage masks

a) Used for dry skin; contain oils, emollients, and humectants; strong moisturizing effect

b) Melted at a little more than body temperature before application: harden to candle like consistency

c) Contain special crystals of gypsum

d) Used for oily and combination skin; generally oil-absorbing and have an exfoliating effect

e) Used for sensitive or dehydrated skin

f) Often seaweed-based

43. A thin, open-meshed fabric of loosely woven cotton is _____.

44. What is the purpose of gauze? _____

_____

45. _____ is sometimes used instead of gauze.

CLIENT CONSULTATION

46. All facial treatments should begin with a _____

47. Why should the record card be kept at hand during the consultation? _____

_____

48. What should the record card contain?

a) _____

b) _____

c) _____

d) _____

_____

e) _____

_____

f) _____

g) _____

h) _____

49. During the consultation, it is important to perform a thorough _____
prior to cleansing.

FACIAL MASSAGE

50. _____ is the manual or mechanical manipulation of the body by rubbing, gently
pinching, kneading, and tapping.

51. What is the purpose of massage? _____

_____

52. Why do cosmetologists perform massage? _____

_____

53. To master massage techniques, you must have a basic knowledge of _____

_____ .

54. Keep hands soft by using _____ and file and shape nails to avoid
_____ your client.

55. The impact of a massage treatment depends on

a) _____

b) _____

c) _____

56. The direction of movement is always from the _____ of the muscle toward its

_____ .

57. Which portion of the muscle is the more movable attachment, meaning it is attached to another muscle or a movable bone or joint? _____

58. Which portion of the muscle is the fixed attachment, meaning it is attached to an immovable section of the skeleton? _____

59. What could result if the muscle is massaged in the wrong direction? _____

_____

60. List the basic massage manipulations:

a) _____

b) _____

c) _____

d) _____

e) _____

f) _____

g) _____

h) _____

i) _____

j) _____

61. Every muscle has a _____ , which is a point on the skin over the muscle where pressure or stimulation will cause contraction of that muscle.

62. Identify the motor points on the illustration below:

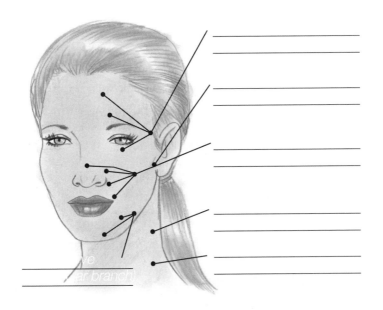

Identify the motor points on the illustration below:

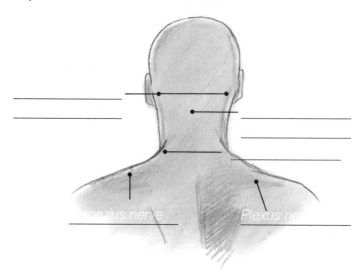

Trapezius nerve   Plexus nerve

63. Relaxation is achieved through _____ or _____

   _____ .

64. The following benefits may be obtained by proper facial and scalp massage:

   a) _____

   b) _____

   c) _____

   d) _____

   e) _____

   f) _____

   g) _____

65. Facial machines will help to

   a) _____

   b) _____

   c) _____

66. A facial _____ heats and produces a stream of warm steam that can be focused
   on the client's face.

67. Steaming the skin helps to _____ , making it more accepting of
   moisturizers and other treatment products. It also helps to _____ follicle
   accumulations such as comedones and clogged follicles.

68. When is steam usually administered? _____

69. A rotating electric appliance with interchangeable brushes that can be attached to a rotating head is a _____

70. Brushing is a form of _____ and is usually administered after or during _____ .

71. What does brushing do? _____

72. Brushing should never be used on clients using _____ _____ or on clients who have _____

73. The skin suction and cold spray machine is used to _____ and to jet-spray lotions and toners onto the skin.

74. Skin suction should only be used on _____ and _____ skin.

ELECTROTHERAPY AND LIGHT THERAPY

75. Galvanic and high frequency treatment is a type of _____ , the use of electrical currents to treat the skin.

76. Electrotherapy should never be administered on

a) _____

b) _____

c) _____

d) _____

e) _____

f) _____

g) _____

77. An _____ is an applicator for directing the electric current from the machine to the client's skin.

78. _____ machines have one electrode, and _____ have two—a positive electrode called an _____ , which has a red plug and cord, and a negative electrode called a _____ , which has a black plug and cord.

79. The process of softening and emulsifying hardened sebum stuck in the follicles is known as _____ .

80. _____ is the process of using galvanic current to penetrate water-soluble products that contain ions into the skin.

81. A type of galvanic treatment that is a computerized device that has many applications in skin care is _____ .

82. _____ current is used to stimulate blood flow and help products penetrate.

83. Electrodes for the high-frequency machine are made of _____ .

84. High frequency can be applied

    a) _____

    b) _____

85. Traditionally, _____ have been used to heat the skin and increase blood flow.

86. What is the newest type of light therapy? _____ .

87. What does this treatment do? _____

88. A type of mechanical exfoliation that uses a closed vacuum to shoot crystals onto the skin, bumping off cell build-up that is then vacuumed by suction, is known as

    _____

FACIAL TREATMENTS

89. Facial treatments fall into two categories:

    a) _____

    b) _____

90. Facial treatments help to

    a) _____

    b) _____

    c) _____

    d) _____

    e) _____

91. Special problems that must be considered when you are performing a facial include

    a) _____

    b) _____

    c) _____

    d) _____

92. What causes dry skin? _____

93. Oily skin is often characterized by _____ , which are caused by hardened masses of sebum formed in the ducts of the sebaceous glands.

94. Acne is a disorder of the _____ that requires thorough and sometimes ongoing medical attention.

95. Generally, medical direction limits the cosmetologists to the following measure in the treatment of acne:

a) _____

b) _____

c) _____

d) _____

96. Because acne skin contains infectious matter, you must wear protective gloves and use disposable materials.

____ True

____ False

97. Home care is probably the most important factor in a successful skin care program. What is the key word in that statement? _____

98. What does a skin care program consist of? _____

_____

AROMATHERAPY

99. Aromatherapy is the therapeutic use of _____ , such as

a) _____

b) _____

c) _____

100. Many essential oils are used for the aromatherapy benefits to enhance a person's

_____

23 FACIAL MAKEUP

Date: _____

Rating: _____

Text Pages: 603-639

POINT TO PONDER:

> *"It's easier to go down the mountain than up, but the view from the top is best."*—**unknown**

1. Makeup is a part of cosmetology that is very interesting and can produce _____ and _____ changes in the appearance.

2. Most clients prefer a _____ , simply covering or focusing attention away from _____ and accenting good facial features.

COSMETICS FOR FACIAL MAKEUP

3. _____ is a tinted cosmetic, also known as _____ , that is used to cover or even out the coloring of the skin.

4. Foundation can be used to _____

5. Foundation is available in _____

6. Most liquid and cream foundations are mixtures of _____ spreading agents as a base containing a significant amount of talc and different coloring agents called

_____

7. Liquid foundations, also called _____ foundations, are mostly water but often contain an emollient such as mineral oil or a silicone such as cyclomethicone.

8. Water-based foundations are most often used for _____ and for oily to _____ skin types.

9. Foundations that are marketed as oil-free are usually intended for _____ .

10. _____ also known as oil-based, are considerably thicker products and are often sold in jars or tins.

11. Cream foundations provide _____ coverage and are usually intended for _____

_____ .

12. What will using cream foundations on oily or acneic skin cause? _____

_____

13. If a cosmetic product causes the formation of clogged pores or comedones, it is called
_____ , which means comedo-producing.

14. Choosing the correct color of foundation is extremely important in _____

_____.

15. Foundation should be as close to the client's _____ as possible.

16. If the foundation is too light, how will it appear? _____

17. If the foundation is too dark, how will it appear? _____

18. What is a line of demarcation? _____

19. _____ foundation contains a lot of pigment for coverage. The pigment
sticks to the skin, providing a natural-looking coverage.

20. _____ are thicker and heavier types of foundation that contain more talc or
pigment for heavier coverage.

21. What are concealers used for?

    a) _____

    b) _____

    c) _____

22. Concealers are not available in a wide range of colors, and it may be difficult to match
skin color.

    ___ True
    ___ False

23. What may happen if concealer color is not matched perfectly to skin tone? _____

_____

24. Some concealers may also contain ingredients to

    a) _____

    b) _____

    c) _____

25. A cosmetic powder that is used to add a matte or nonshiny finish to the face is a

_____.

26. Face powder

   a) _____

   b) _____

   c) _____

27. Face powder is available in two forms: _____

28. Pressed powder is blended with a _____ to keep it in a caked form in the tin. _____ does not contain as much binder and comes in a jar.

29. Should powder puffs ever be used in the salon? Why? _____

30. What is the purpose of cheek color? _____

_____

31. What forms does cheek color come in? _____

32. _____ is a paste-like cosmetic, usually in a metal or plastic tube, available in a large variety of colors and used to change or enhance the color of the lips.

33. Some lip color products contain conditioners to moisturize the lips or sunscreen to protect against sun exposure.

   ____ True

   ____ False

34. Lip color is available in a variety of forms including _____ and _____.

35. Lip color must blend with the client's _____ and other makeup used.

36. _____ is a colored pencil used to outline the lips and keep the lipstick from bleeding into small lines around the mouth.

37. Lip liner is usually applied before the lip color to _____.

38. How do you choose the lip liner color? _____

_____

39. _____ are cosmetics applied on the eyelids to accentuate or contour them.

40. Eye shadows are available in a variety of finishes, including

   a) _____

   b) _____

c) _____

d) _____

e) _____

41. Eye shadows are available in:

    a) _____

    b) _____

    c) _____

    d) _____

42. Match each of the following eye shadows with its description:

    ___ 1. Base color   a) A shade lighter than the client's skin tone used to make an area appear larger

    ___ 2. Contour color   b) A medium tone close to the client's skin tone

    ___ 3. Highlight color   c) Deeper and darker than the client's skin tone

43. _____ is a cosmetic used to outline and emphasize the eyes.

44. Eyeliner is available in a variety of colors, in pencil, _____ , pressed, or felt tip pen form.

45. What does eyeliner do? _____

46. Eyeliner pencils consist of a wax _____ or hardened oil base _____ with a variety of additives to create color.

47. _____ are used to add color and shape to the eyebrows, usually after tweezing or waxing.

48. _____ is a cosmetic preparation used to darken, define, and thicken the eyelashes.

49. Mascara is available in _____ .

50. _____ remove eye makeup products that are water-resistant.

51. _____ is a heavy makeup used for theatrical purposes.

52. A shaped, solid mass applied to the face with a moistened cosmetic sponge is

_____

MAKEUP COLOR THEORY

53. _____ are fundamental colors that cannot be obtained from a mixture.

54. _____ are obtained by mixing equal parts of two primary colors.

55. _____ are obtained by mixing equal amounts of a secondary color and its neighboring primary color on the color wheel.

56. The primary colors are: _____ , and _____

57. A primary and secondary color directly opposite each other on the color wheel are called

_____ .

58. When mixed, complementary colors cancel each other out to create a _____ _____ color.

59. _____ are the range of colors from yellow and gold through the oranges, red-oranges, most reds, and even some yellow-greens.

60. _____ suggest coolness and are dominated by blues, greens, violets, and blue-reds.

BASIC MAKEUP APPLICATION

61. The first step in the makeup process is the _____

62. You should _____ and try not to impose your own opinions too much.

63. The consultation area must be _____

64. Describe the type of lighting that is required for a makeup consultation area: _____

_____

_____

65. What information should you record on the consultation card?

a) _____

b) _____

c) _____

d) _____

e) _____

f) _____

CORRECTIVE MAKEUP

66. Creative makeup techniques are used to _____
_____

67. Facial features can be _____ with proper highlighting, _____ with correct shadowing or shading, and _____ with the proper hairstyle.

68. The basic rule of makeup application is to _____
_____

ARTIFICIAL EYELASHES

69. Why has the use of artificial eyelashes grown enormously?

   a) _____

   b) _____

70. What is the objective of artificial eyelashes? _____
_____

71. _____ , also called strip lashes, are eyelash hairs on a strip that are applied with adhesive to the natural lash line.

72. _____ are separate artificial eyelashes that are applied to the eyelids one at a time.

73. _____ is the product used to make artificial eyelashes adhere to the natural lash line.

24 NAIL DISEASES & DISORDERS

Date:
_____

Rating:
_____

Text Pages: 641-654

POINT TO PONDER:

> *"Many things will catch your eye, but only a few will catch your heart . . .*
> *pursue those."*—*unknown*

1. Describe a normal healthy nail: _____

2. Certain health problems in the body can show up in the nails as visible disorders or poor nail growth.

   ___ True

   ___ False

NAIL DISORDERS

3. A _____ is a condition caused by injury or disease.

4. You can help your clients with nail disorders in one of two ways.

   a) _____

   b) _____

5. When should a client not receive services? _____
   _____ What should you do if any of these are present? _____
   _____

6. _____ are a condition in which a blood clot forms under the nail plate, forming a dark purplish spot.

7. _____ run vertically down the length of the natural nail plate and are caused by _____ of the nails, usually the result of _____

8. What can be done to minimize the appearance of ridges?

   a) _____

   b) _____

9. A noticeably thin, white nail plate that is much more flexible than normal is known as an

_____ .

10. What conditions usually cause eggshell nails? _____

_____

11. Why should heavy pressure with a pusher not be used at the base of eggshell nails?

_____

12. Visible depressions running across the width of the natural nail plate are _____

They usually result from _____ or _____ that has traumatized the body.

13. A _____ or agnail is a condition in which the living skin splits around the nail.

14. What will aid in correcting hangnails? _____

15. White spots, or _____ spots, are a whitish discoloration of the nails, usually

caused by injury to the nail matrix.

16. The darkening of the fingernails or toenails is _____ .

17. _____ , or bitten nails, is the result of a habit that promotes the individual to

chew the nail or the hardened, damage skin surrounding the nail plate.

18. The condition of split or brittle nails that also have a series of lengthwise ridges giving a

rough appearance to the surface of the nail plate is _____

19. This condition is usually caused by

a) _____

b) _____

c) _____

d) _____

e) _____

f) _____

20. Plicatured nail literally means _____ and is a type of highly curved nail plate

often caused by injury to the _____ , but it may be _____ .

21. An abnormal condition that occurs when skin is stretched by the nail plate is nail

_____

22. The terms "cuticle" and "pterygium" are the same thing and may be used interchangeably.

____ True

____ False

23. Nail pterygium is abnormal damage to the _____ or _____ and should not be treated by pushing the extension of skin back with an instrument.

24. Explain the proper way to care for pterygium: _____

_____

25. Nail plates with a deep or sharp curvature at the free edge have this shape because of the _____ . This is known as a _____ .

26. _____ are parasites that under some circumstances may cause infections of the feet and hands.

27. Why is nail fungi of concern to the salon? _____

_____

28. How can the transmission of fungal infections be avoided? _____

_____

29. In the past, discolorations of the nail plate were incorrectly referred to as _____ .

30. The discoloration is a bacterial infection caused by one of several types of _____ .

NAIL DISEASES

31. Are there any nail diseases that should be treated in the salon?

____ Yes

____ No

32. Match each of the following nail diseases with its description:

_____ 1. Onychosis

_____ 2. Onychia

_____ 3. Onychocryptosis

_____ 4. Onycholysis

_____ 5. Onychomadesis

_____ 6. Nail psoriasis

_____ 7. Paronychia

_____ 8. Pyogenic granuloma

_____ 9. Tinea pedis

_____ 10. Onychomycosis

a) Ingrown nails

b) The separation and falling off of a nail plate from the nail bed

c) A bacterial inflammation of the tissues surrounding the nail

d) The medical term for fungal infections of the feet

e) A severe inflammation of the nail in which a lump of red tissue grows up from the nail bed to the nail plate

f) Any deformity or disease of the nail

g) the lifting of the nail plate from the bed without shedding

h) A fungal infection of the nail plate

i) Tiny pits or severe roughness on the surface of the nail plate

j) An inflammation of the nail matrix followed by the shedding of the natural nail plate

25 MANICURING

See Milady's Standard Cosmetology Practical Workbook

26 PEDICURING

See Milady's Standard Cosmetology Practical Workbook

27 NAIL TIPS, WRAPS, & NO LIGHT GELS

See Milady's Standard Cosmetology Practical Workbook

28 ACRYLIC (METHACRYLATE) NAILS

See Milady's Standard Cosmetology Practical Workbook

29 UV GELS

See Milady's Standard Cosmetology Practical Workbook

30 SEEKING EMPLOYMENT

Date: _____

Rating: _____

Text Pages: 790-818

POINT TO PONDER:

"The ability to concentrate and to use your time well is everything."
—Lee Iacocca

PREPARING FOR LICENSURE

1. List the factors that will affect how well you perform during the licensing examination or on tests in general:

   a) _____

   b) _____

   c) _____

   d) _____

   e) _____

2. Being _____ means understanding the _____ for successfully taking tests.

3. A test-wise student prepares for taking a test by practicing _____ and
   _____.

4. List the daily habits and time management skills of effective studying:

   a) _____

   b) _____

   c) _____

   d) _____

   e) _____

   f) _____

   g) _____

   h) _____

5. What holistic steps can you take to prepare for test taking?

a) _____

b) _____

c) _____

d) _____

e) _____

6. What strategies can you adapt on test day?

a) _____

b) _____

c) _____

d) _____

e) _____

f) _____

g) _____
_____

h) _____

i) _____
_____

j) _____
_____

k) _____

l) _____
_____

m) _____
_____

n) _____
_____

o) _____

p) _____
_____

7. _____ is the process of reaching logical conclusions by employing logical reasoning.

8. When taking a test, you should begin by eliminating options you know are incorrect.

    ___ True
    ___ False

9. Study the _____ , or the _____ , it will often provide a clue to the correct answer.

10. In reading type tests that contain long paragraphs followed by several questions, read the _____ first. This will help identify the _____ elements in the paragraph.

11. The most important strategy of test taking is to _____.

12. In true/false questions look for qualifying words such as _____
    _____ absolutes are generally _____

13. In a true/false statement, only part of the statement needs to be true.

    ___ True
    ___ False

14. When taking a multiple choice test, read the entire question carefully, including all the
    _____.

15. When answering multiple choice questions, it is wise to eliminate completely incorrect answers first.

    ___ True
    ___ False

16. When answering matching questions, it is best to read all items in each list before beginning.

    ___ True
    ___ False

17. When answering essay questions, make sure that what you write is _____
    _____ , and _____.

18. To be successful at test taking, you must follow the rules of _____ and be _____ of the exam content for both the practical and written examination.

19. To be better prepared for the practical portion of the exam, the new graduate will:

a) _____

b) _____
_____

c) _____
_____

d) _____
_____

e) _____
_____

f) _____

g) _____
_____

h) _____

i) _____

PREPARING FOR EMPLOYMENT

20. Answer the following questions:

a) What do you really want out of a career in cosmetology? _____
_____

b) What particular areas within the beauty industry interests you most? _____
_____

c) What are your strongest practical skills, and in what ways do you wish to use them?
_____

d) What personal qualities will help you have a successful career? _____
_____

21. Willingness to work hard is a key ingredient to your _____

22. List the key personal characteristics that will help you get and keep the position you want:

a) _____

b) _____

c) _____

d) _____

e) _____

23. Match the following type of salon with the phrase that best describes it:

____ 1. Small independent salon

____ 2. Independent salon chain

____ 3. Large national salon chain

____ 4. Franchise salon

a) Chains of five or more salons that are owned by one individual

b) Chain salon organization, one with a national name, owned by individuals who pay a fee to use the name

c) Salon owned by an individual or two or more partners

d) Company operates salons throughout the country

24. Match the following type of salon with the phrase that best describes it:

____ 1. Value priced salon

____ 2. Full-service salons

____ 3. Image salons

a) Salons that offer luxurious, higher-priced services and treatments

b) Salons that depend on high volume of traffic and charge low prices

c) Salons that offer a complete menu of hair, nail, and skin care services

25. What is possibly the least expensive way of owning one's own business? _____

26. When preparing your professional resume follow these guidelines:

a) _____

b) _____

c) _____
   _____

d) _____

e) _____
   _____

f) _____

g) _____

27. The average potential employer will spend _____ scanning your resume before deciding whether or not to grant you an interview.

28. When writing a resume, you should focus on your _____.

29. List the do's and don'ts of resumes:

DO's

    a) _____

    b) _____

    c) _____

    d) _____

    e) _____

    f) _____

    g) _____

    h) _____

DON'TS

    i) _____

    j) _____

    k) _____

    l) _____

30. An _____ is a collection of photos and documents that reflect your skills, accomplishments, and abilities in your chosen career.

31. A powerful portfolio includes

    a) _____

    b) _____

    c) _____

    d) _____

    e) _____

    f) _____

    g) _____

h) _____

i) _____

j) _____

32. List the points to consider when narrowing your job search for the best possible results:

a) _____

b) _____

c) _____

d) _____

e) _____

33. A great way to find out about jobs is to actually _____

34. _____ allows you to establish contacts that may eventually lead to a job and helps you gain valuable information about the workings of various establishments.

35. List the guidelines to follow when networking with local salons:

a) _____

b) _____

c) _____
   _____

d) _____
   _____

e) _____
   _____

f) _____
   _____

36. When you visit the salon, take your _____ to ensure that you observe all the key areas that might affect your decision making.

37. After visiting a salon, remember to _____
   _____

38. When you decide to make contact with an appropriate salon to ask for an interview, you should send your resume only.

_____ True

_____ False

39. When preparing for an interview, make sure you have all the following items in place:

a) _____

b) _____

c) _____

d) _____

e) _____

40. What supporting materials should you also have in place?

a) _____

b) _____

c) _____

41. The following questions are typical of the ones you may be asked during an interview. To prepare yourself for the interview, answer the questions now.

a) What did you like best about your training? _____
_____
_____

b) Are you punctual and regular in attendance? _____
_____
_____

c) Will your school director or instructor confirm this? _____
_____
_____

d) What skills do you feel are your strongest? _____
_____
_____

e) What areas do you consider to be less strong? _____
_____
_____

f) Are you a team player? Please explain. _____

_____

_____

g) Do you consider yourself flexible? Please explain. _____

_____

_____

h) What are your career goals? _____

_____

i) What days and hours are you available for work? _____

_____

_____

j) Do you have your own transportation? _____

_____

_____

k) Are there any obstacles that would prevent you from keeping your commitment to full time employment? _____

_____

l) What assets do you believe that you would bring to this salon and this position? _____

_____

_____

m) Who is the most interesting person you have met in your work and/or education experience? _____

_____

_____

n) How would you handle a problem client? _____

_____

_____

o) How do you feel about retailing? _____

_____

_____

p) Would you be willing to attend our company training program? _____

_____

_____

q) Describe ways that you provide excellent customer service: _____

_____

_____

r) Please share an example of consultation questions that you might ask a client. _____

_____

_____

s) What steps do you take to build your business and ensure that clients return to see you?

_____

_____

42. What behaviors should you practice in connection with the interview?

a) _____

b) _____

c) _____

d) _____

e) _____

f) _____

g) _____

h) _____

i) _____

j) _____

k) _____

l) _____

43. List some questions that you might consider asking during a job interview:

a) _____

b) _____

c) _____

d) _____

e) _____

f) _____

g) _____

h) _____

i) _____

_____

j) _____

k) _____

l) _____

44. Next to each question, indicate whether it is legal or illegal to be asked it in an interview:

a) How old are you?   _____

b) Would you describe your medical history?   _____

c) Are you over the age of 18?   _____

d) Are you able to perform this job?   _____

e) Are you a U.S. citizen?   _____

f) Are you authorized to work in the United States?   _____

g) In which languages are you fluent?   _____

45. Once employed, take the necessary steps to learn all you can about your new position by

a) _____

b) _____

c) _____

31 ON THE JOB

Date: _____

Rating: _____

Text Pages: 819-838

POINT TO PONDER:

> *"You cannot always have happiness, but you can always give happiness."*
> —unknown

MOVING FROM SCHOOL TO WORK

1. One you become the employee of a salon, you are expected to put the needs of the _____ ahead of your own.

2. Putting the salon and the clients needs first means

   a) _____

   b) _____

OUT IN THE REAL WORLD

3. In a job, you will never have to do any work or perform services that aren't what you want to do.

   ____ True

   ____ False

4. To be successful, you must determine the position that is _____

5. The number one thing to remember when you are in a service business is that your work revolves around _____.

6. List the key points to remember in serving others.

   a) _____

   b) _____

   c) _____

   d) _____

e) _____

f) _____

g) _____

7. Working in a salon requires that you practice and perfect your _____ and become a good _____.

8. List the habits of successful team players:

a) _____

b) _____

c) _____

d) _____

e) _____

f) _____

g) _____

h) _____

9. When you take a job, you will be expected to

a) _____

b) _____

c) _____

10. A document that outlines all the duties and responsibilities of a particular position in a salon or spa is a _____

11. If your salon does not have a job description, you may want to _____

12. If you are unclear about something, you should _____.

13. A job description should cover

a) _____

b) _____

c) _____

14. The three standard methods of compensation in a salon are _____ and _____.

15. A salaried position is generally offered to a new practitioner and is usually based on

_____ .

16. A _____ a percentage of the revenue that the salon takes in from its sales, is usually offered to practitioners once they have built up a loyal clientele.

17. Commissions are paid on your total _____ .

18. Commissions range anywhere from 25% to 60% and is usually based on:

a) _____

b) _____

c) _____

19. A salary-plus-commission structure basically means that you receive both a _____ and a _____

20. This kind of structure is commonly used to _____ practitioners to perform more services.

21. It is customary for salon professionals to receive _____ from satisfied clients.

22. Tips must be reported as income.

____ True

____ False

23. An _____ is the best way to keep tabs on your progress and to get feedback from your salon manager and key coworkers.

24. Commonly, evaluations are scheduled _____ days after hiring and then once a year after that.

25. Ask a _____ to sit in on one of your client consultations and make note of areas where you can improve.

26. One of the best ways to improve your performance is to model your behavior after someone who is having the kind of success you wish to have and to use that person as a

_____ .

27. When seeking out a role model, observe the stylist who is really good and determine

a) _____

b) _____

c) _____

d) _____

e) _____

f) _____

g) _____

MANAGING YOUR MONEY

28. A career in the beauty industry is very _____ ; it is also a career that requires _____ and planning.

29. The best way to meet all of your financial responsibilities is to know _____ , so you can make informed decisions about where your money goes.

30. Keeping track of where your money goes is _____ _____ .

31. How can you generate greater income for yourself?

a) _____

b) _____

c) _____

32. To get help with personal finances, you should seek the advice of a personal _____ , who will be able to give you advice on reducing your credit card debt, investing your money, and retirement options.

DISCOVER THE SELLING YOU

33. The practice of recommending and selling additional services to your clients is called _____ or _____ .

34. _____ is the act of recommending and selling products to your clients for at home hair, skin, and nail care.

35. To be successful in sales, you need

a) _____

b) _____

c) _____

36. What is the first step in selling? _____

37. List the principles of selling

a) _____

b) _____

c) _____

d) _____

e) _____

f) _____

_____

g) _____

_____

h) _____

38. A _____ involves informing the client about the product, without stressing they purchase it. A _____ approach focuses emphatically on why a client should buy the product.

39. What are the various reasons clients are motivated to buying salon products?

a) _____

b) _____

c) _____

40. Your first consideration is to always keep in mind the _____.

41. How can you get the conversation started on retailing products?

a) _____

_____

b) _____

c) _____

_____

d) _____

e) _____

f) _____

_____

42. Once you have mastered the basics of good service, take a look at some _____ _____ that will keep your clients coming back to you.

43. List suggested marketing techniques that will keep your clients coming back to you:

a) _____

b) _____

c) _____

d) _____

44. What things can you do to build your client base?

a) _____

b) _____

c) _____

d) _____

e) _____

45. The best time to think about getting your client back into the salon is while she is still in your salon.

____ True

____ False

46. The best way to encourage your client to book another appointment before she leaves is to _____ .

32 THE SALON BUSINESS

Date: _____

Rating: _____

Text Pages: 839-860

POINT TO PONDER:

> *"He who does not get fun and enjoyment out of every day . . . needs to reorganize his life."*—**George Matthew Adams**

GOING INTO BUSINESS FOR YOURSELF

1. The two main options for being your own boss are

   a) _____

   b) _____

2. In a booth rental arrangement, a practitioner generally

   a) _____

   b) _____

   c) _____

   d) _____

   e) _____

3. Booth rental is a desirable situation for _____

   _____

4. What are the obligations of renting a booth?

   a) _____

   b) _____

   c) _____

   d) _____

   e) _____

f) _____

g) _____

h) _____

_____

5. As a booth renter, you will not enjoy the same benefits as an employee of a salon would, such as _____

6. List the basic factors to carefully consider when opening a salon.

a) _____

b) _____

c) _____

d) _____

e) _____

f) _____

g) _____

7. What are the elements of a good business location? _____

_____

8. A _____ is a written description of your business as you see it today and as you foresee it in the next 5 years.

9. What should be included in your business plan?

a) _____

b) _____

c) _____

d) _____

e) _____

10. What is meant by area demographics? _____

_____

11. What kind of laws must be complied with when you open a salon? _____

_____

12. What kind of insurance must be purchased when you open your business? _____

_____

13. What are the three types of ownership?

    a) _____

    b) _____

    c) _____

14. Describe a business that is owned by a sole proprietor: _____

_____

_____

15. Describe a partnership: _____

_____

_____

16. Describe a business owned by a corporation: _____

_____

_____

17. If you choose to purchase an existing salon, your agreement to purchase should include:

    a) _____

    b) _____

    _____

    c) _____

    _____

    d) _____

    e) _____

    f) _____

    _____

    g) _____

    _____

18. A lease should specify the following:

    a) _____

    _____

    b) _____

    _____

c) _____

19. What can you do to protect the salon against fire, theft, and lawsuits?

    a) _____

    _____

    b) _____

    _____

    c) _____

    _____

    d) _____

    _____

    _____

20. To run a people oriented business you need

    a) _____

    b) _____

21. Smooth business management depends on the following factors:

    a) _____

    b) _____

    c) _____

    d) _____

    e) _____

    f) _____

    g) _____

22. As a business operator, you must always know where your money _____ .

23. Proper _____ are necessary to meet the needs of local, state, and federal laws regarding taxes and employees.

24. _____ is classified as receipts from service and retail sales.

25. _____ include rent, utilities, insurance, salaries, advertising, equipment, and repairs.

26. _____ help establish the net worth of the business at the end of the year.

27. Supplies that are used in the daily business operation are _____ and those to be sold to clients are _____ .

OPERATING A SUCCESSFUL SALON

28. How can you ensure that you will stay in business and have a prosperous salon?

_____

29. When planning the salon's layout, maximum _____ should be the primary concern.

30. The retail area should be spacious, _____ and well lit.

31. What determines the number of salon employees? _____

32. When interviewing potential employees, consider the following:

a) _____

b) _____

c) _____

d) _____

e) _____

33. What are some ways you can share your success with your staff?

a) _____

b) _____

c) _____

d) _____

e) _____

f) _____

_____

g) _____

34. The best salons employ professional _____ to handle the job of scheduling appointments and greeting clients.

35. The reception area should be _____

36. A well-trained receptionist is the _____ of the salon.

37. The receptionist should be _____

_____ .

38. The receptionist handles important functions such as

a) _____

b) _____

c) _____

d) _____

e) _____

39. Appointments must be scheduled to make the most efficient use of everyone's _____ .

40. The receptionist must have the following qualities:

a) _____

b) _____

c) _____

41. The appointment book may be an actual book that sits atop the reception desk, or it may be a _____ appointment book.

42. An important part of the salon business is handled over the _____ .

43. When using the telephone you should

a) _____

_____

b) _____

c) _____

_____

d) _____

44. Incoming phone calls are the _____ of the salon.

45. When booking appointments what information should you ask? _____

_____

46. If the practitioner is not available when the client requests, what ways can this situation be handled?

a) _____

b) _____

c) _____

_____

47. When handling complaints over the phone, how should you respond? _____

_____

48. The tone of your voice must be _____ and _____.

49. What is advertising? _____

50. Advertising must _____

_____

51. What is the best form of advertising? _____

52. What kind of advertising venues are available?

a) _____

b) _____

c) _____

d) _____

e) _____

f) _____

_____

g) _____

h) _____

i) _____

j) _____

_____

k) _____

l) _____

m) _____

_____

n) _____

53. An important aspect of the salon's financial success revolves around the sale of

_____ .

TEST I: MULTIPLE CHOICE TEST

Directions: Carefully read each statement. Circle the word or phrase that correctly completes the statement.

1. Kosmetikos is a Greek word meaning_____ .

   a) Skilled in haircare

   b) Skilled in the study of cosmetics

   c) Licensed cosmetologist

   d) Licensed barber

2. In ancient cultures, the practice of self-grooming and appearance enhancement was allied with the practice of _____ .

   a) Dentistry

   b) Medicine

   c) Barbers

   d) Priests

3. The two types of goals are _____ .

   a) Daily and yearly

   b) Short-term and life

   c) Daily and long-term

   d) Short-term and long-term

4. Comfortable well-fitted shoes should have _____ .

   a) Low heels

   b) Chunky heels

   c) Narrow heels

   d) Pointed toes

5. Verbal communication with a client to determine desired results is _____ .

   a) Clarification

   b) Communication

   c) Client consultation

   d) Reflective listening

6. An agency created as part of the Department of Labor to regulate and enforce safety and health standards to protect the employee in the workplace is _____ .

   a) MSDS

   b) OSHA

   c) State Board

   d) EPA

7. An infectious microorganism capable of infesting almost all plants and animals is

   _____ .

   a) Bacteria

   b) Virus

   c) Toxin

   d) Parasite

8. Bacteria that are completely harmless and do not cause disease are _____ .

   a) Microbes

   b) Germs

   c) Nonpathogenic

   d) Pathogenic

9. The virus that causes AIDS is _____ .

   a) EPA

   b) MSD

   c) HIV

   d) QUATS

10. Agents that are formulated for use on skin are _____.

   a) Disinfectants

   b) Antiseptics

   c) Sterilizers

   d) Sanitizers

11. _____ acts like a balloon to contain the protoplasm.

   a) Cell membrane

   b) Cytoplasm

   c) Metabolism

   d) Anabolism

12. The physical foundation of the body is the _____ system.

   a) Muscular

   b) Skeletal

   c) Circulatory

   d) Nervous

13. The sides of the head in the ear region is formed by the _____

   a) Parietal bone

   b) Occipital bone

   c) Frontal bone

   d) Temporal bone

14. The uppermost and largest bone of the arm is the _____.

   a) Ulna

   b) Radius

   c) Carpus

   d) Humerus

15. The tendon that connects the occipitalis and the frontalis is the _____.

   a) Aponeurosis

   b) Epicranius

   c) Masseter

   d) Platysma

16. The _____ nerve affects the skin of the forehead, scalp, eyebrow, and upper eyelid.

   a) Infratrochlear

   b) Auriculotemporal

   c) Infraorbital

   d) Superorbital

17. The _____ is also called the gastrointestinal system and is responsible for breaking down food into nutrients and waste.

   a) Endocrine

   b) Digestive

   c) Excretory

   d) Respiratory

18. The basal cell layer, composed of several layers of different shaped cells, is the

   _____ .

   a) Stratum lucidum

   b) Stratum granulosum

   c) Stratum corneum

   d) Stratum germinativum

19. What controls the excretion of sweat? _____

   a) Circulatory system

   b) Respiratory system

   c) Nervous system

   d) Excretory system

20. Vitamin _____ is an antioxidant that can help prevent certain types of cancers.

    a) A

    b) B

    c) C

    d) D

21. _____ supplies nutrients and oxygen to the skin.

    a) Lymph

    b) Blood

    c) Nerves

    d) Sweat

22. The nail bed is supplied with many nerves and is attached to the nail plate by a thin layer of tissue called the _____.

    a) Hyponychium

    b) Epoynichium

    c) Bed epithelium

    d) Nail grooves

23. The _____ is the living skin at the base of the nail plate covering the matrix area.

    a) Hyponychium

    b) Epoynichium

    c) Bed epithelium

    d) Nail grooves

24. The hardened keratin plate covering the nail bed is the _____.

    a) Nail groove

    b) Nail fold

    c) Nail plate

    d) Nail bed

25. A mature strand of human hair is divided into two parts: the root and the _____.

    a) Hair bulb

    b) Dermal papilla

    c) Follicle

    d) Hair shaft

26. A chemical side bond that is very different from the physical bond of hydrogen or salt bonds is a _____ bond.

    a) Cysteine

    b) Side

    c) Disulfide

    d) Hydrogen

27. The growth phase of the hair is the _____ phase.

    a) Anagen

    b) Catagen

    c) Telogen

    d) Vellus

28. The medical term for dandruff is _____.

    a) Hypertrichosis

    b) Monilet

    c) Canities

    d) Pityriasis

29. _____ is a condition of abnormal growth of hair.

    a) Hypertrichosis

    b) Trichoptilosis

    c) Trichorrhexis nodosa

    d) Fragilitas crinium

30. A _____ is a stable mixture of two or mixable substances.

    a) Solute

    b) Solution

    c) Solvent

    d) Suspension

31. A sweet, colorless, oily substance is _____.

    a) Ammonia

    b) Glycerin

    c) Alkanolamines

    d) Compound

32. A chemical reaction that easily transmits heat is called _____.

    a) Oxidation

    b) Combustion

    c) Exothermic

    d) Endothermic

33. A/an _____ is any substance that conducts electricity.

    a) Current

    b) Conductor

    c) Insulator

    d) Circuit

34. A unit that measures the strength of an electric current is a/an _____.

    a) Volt

    b) Amp

    c) Ohm

    d) Watt

35. The _____ current is a thermal or heat producing current with a high rate of oscillation or vibration.

    a) Galvanic

    b) Faradic

    c) Sinusoidal

    d) Tesla-high frequency

36. _____ forces acidic substances into deeper tissues using galvanic current from the positive toward the negative poles.

    a) Cataphoresis

    b) Anaphoresis

    c) Iontophoresis

    d) Disincrustation

37. Lines that are parallel to the floor are _____.

    a) Vertical

    b) Horizontal

    c) Diagonal

    d) Curved

38. Curved lines used to soften and blend horizontal or vertical lines are known as _____.

    a) Single line

    b) Transitional line

    c) Contrasting line

    d) Repeating line

39. The five principles of hair design are proportion, rhythm, emphasis, harmony, and _____.

    a) Symmetry

    b) Asymmetry

    c) Diagonal

    d) Balance

40. Generally the ideal face shape is the _____ shape.

    a) Square

    b) Triangle

    c) Oval

    d) Pear

41. The _____ part should be used to create width or height in a hairstyle.

    a) Triangular

    b) Side

    c) Zigzag

    d) Diagonal

42. A process that lightens and colors hair in a single application is known as

    _____.

    a) Double-process haircoloring

    b) Temporary rinsing

    c) Virgin haircoloring

    d) Single-process haircoloring

43. Haircolor that is mixed with a developer and remains in the hair shaft until the new
    growth of hair occurs is called _____.

    a) Temporary

    b) Semipermanent

    c) Demipermanent

    d) Permanent

44. The cortex or middle layer of the hair gives strength and elasticity and contributes about
    _____ % to the overall strength of the hair.

    a) 10

    b) 20

    c) 50

    d) 80

45. The free-form technique of hair painting is also called _____ .

    a) Toning

    b) Baliage

    c) Brushing

    d) Swabbing

46. The two methods of parting hair for a foil technique are _____ .

    a) Slicing and striping

    b) Weaving and striping

    c) Slicing and threading

    d) Slicing and weaving

47. The haircolor that partially penetrates the hair shaft and stains the cuticle layer, slowly fading with each shampoo is known as _____ .

    a) Temporary

    b) Semipermanent

    c) Demipermanent

    d) Permanent

48. An itchy, swollen lesion that lasts only a few hours is a _____ .

    a) Tubercle

    b) Wheal

    c) Bulla

    d) Macule

49. A skin condition caused by an inflammation of the sebaceous glands is _____ .

    a) Asteatosis

    b) Seborrheic dermatitis

    c) Steatoma

    d) Rosacea

50. An abnormal growth of skin is called ________________.

a) Hypertrichosis

b) Hypertrophy

c) Kertoma

d) Callus

51. An abnormal brown or wine-colored skin discoloration with a circular and irregular shape is called a ________________.

a) Macule

b) Skin tag

c) Mole

d) Stain

52. A fungal infection of the natural nail plate is ________________.

a) Onychocryptosis

b) Onychia

c) Onychophagy

d) Onychomycosis

53. Severe inflammation of the nail in which a lump of red tissue grows up from the nail bed to the nail plate is a ________________.

a) Plicatured nail

b) Pyogenic granuloma

c) Pincer nail

d) Tinea pedis

54. Noticeably thin, white nail plate that is more flexible than normal is a (e ________________.

a) Eggshell nail

b) Bruised nail

c) Melanonychia

d) Nail pterygium

55. The _____ is the highest point on the head.

    a) Occipital

    b) Apex

    c) Parietal ridge

    d) Four corners

56. The tool used to remove bulk from the hair is called _____.

    a) Haircutting shear

    b) Thinning shear

    c) Clipper

    d) Trimmers

57. A one length haircut is called a _____.

    a) Blunt cut

    b) Graduate cut

    c) Layered cut

    d) Long layered cut

58. The process of thinning the hair to graduated lengths with shears is _____.

    a) Notching

    b) Free-hand notching

    c) Slithering

    d) Point cutting

59. The process of shaping and directing the hair into an s pattern with the use of fingers, combs, and waving lotion is _____.

    a) Pincurls

    b) Fingerwaves

    c) Roller sets

    d) Carved curls

60. A _____ curl permits medium movement.

   a) No stem

   b) Half stem

   c) Full stem

   d) Over stem

61. _____ are used to create height in the hair design.

   a) Barrel curls

   b) Carved curls

   c) Cascade curls

   d) Ridge curls

62. _____ brushes are used to speed up the blow drying process.

   a) Paddle

   b) Vent

   c) Round

   d) Grooming

63. _____ adds considerable weight to the hair by causing strands to join together.

   a) Gel

   b) Mousse

   c) Pomade

   d) Volumizer

64. _____ give a finished appearance to hair ends.

   a) End curls

   b) Volume thermal curls

   c) Volume base curls

   d) Full base curls

65. A board of fine, upright nails through which human hair extensions are combed is a

    _____ .

    a) Hackle

    b) Drawing

    c) Extension

    d) Drafting

66. _____ are narrow rows of visible braids that lie close to the scalp.

    a) Cornrow

    b) Single

    c) Visible

    d) Locks

67. Wigs that are constructed with a combination of synthetic hair and hand-tied human hair

    are _____ .

    a) Hand-knotted

    b) Semi-hand-tied

    c) Machine made

    d) Wefts

68. The removal of hair by means of an electric current that destroys the growth cell of the

    hair is _____ .

    a) Photo-epilation

    b) Electrolysis

    c) Laser

    d) Sugaring

69. A/an _____ removes the hair by removing it from the bottom of the follicle.

    a) Epilator

    b) Depilatory

    c) Tweezer

    d) Thread

70. _____ bonds are chemical side bonds formed when the sulfur atoms in two adjacent protein chains are joined together.

   a) Disulfide

   b) Salt

   c) Hydrogen

   d) Peptide

71. Perm rods that are equal in diameter along their entire length and produce a uniform curl along the entire width of the strand are _____ .

   a) Concave rods

   b) Straight rods

   c) Soft bender rods

   d) Loop rods

72. With a colorless liquid with a strong unpleasant odor, _____ is the most common reducing agent.

   a) Thioglycolic acid

   b) Ammonium thioglycolate

   c) Glyceryl monothioglycolate

   d) True acid

73. The perm wrap where hair is wrapped at an angle other than perpendicular to the length of the rod, and produces a uniform curl from the scalp to the ends is the _____ .

   a) Basic perm wrap

   b) Curvature perm wrap

   c) Bricklay wrap

   d) Spiral wrap

74. _____ relaxers are usually advertised and sold as "no lye" relaxer, containing two components that must be mixed immediately prior to use.

   a) Metal hydroxide

   b) Sodium hydroxide

   c) Guanidine relaxer

   d) Lithium hydroxide

75. Skin with obvious large pores with a shiny, thick appearance is _____ .

   a) Oily skin

   b) Dry skin

   c) Combination

   d) Acne

76. _____ are products that help remove excess dead cells from the skin surface.

   a) Toners

   b) Cleansers

   c) Enzyme peels

   d) Exfoliants

77. _____ is a light, continuous stroking movement applied with the fingers or the palms in a slow rhythmic manner.

   a) Petrissage

   b) Effleurage

   c) Friction

   d) Tapotement

78. A thicker and heavier type of foundation that contain more talc or pigment for heavier coverage are _____ .

   a) Concealers

   b) Powders

   c) Base

   d) Blush

79. The complimentary color for green eyes is _____ .

   a) Blue

   b) Red

   c) Yellow

   d) Green

80. _____ eyes can be lengthened by extending the shadow beyond the outer corner of the eyes.

    a) Round

    b) Close set

    c) Wide set

    d) Heavy lidded

81. _____ brush is a comb-like brush used to remove excess mascara on lashes or to comb brows into place.

    a) Eyeliner

    b) Lash and brow

    c) Powder

    d) Eye shadow

82. _____ are designed to loosen and dissolve dead tissue from the nail plate so that it can be more easily and thoroughly removed.

    a) Cuticle remover

    b) Cream remover

    c) Nail bleach

    d) Pumice powder

83. _____ contain ingredients to reduce brittleness of the nail plate and moisturize the surrounding skin.

    a) Top coat

    b) Base coat

    c) Nail hardener

    d) Nail conditioner

84. A/an _____ involves deep rubbing to the muscles.

    a) Friction movement

    b) Effleurage

    c) Kneading movement

    d) Petrissage

85. A product containing softening agents or oils to penetrate dry, flaky skin and calluses that need to be smoothed during a pedicure is _____ .

   a) Abrasive scrub

   b) Callus softener

   c) Paraffin wax

   d) Foot soak

86. A _____ is used to exfoliate dry skin or smooth calluses.

   a) Nail file

   b) Nail rasp

   c) Foot file

   d) Nippers

87. _____ is a closely woven, heavy material that is opaque, even after adhesive is applied:

   a) Silk

   b) Fiberglas

   c) Fabric

   d) Linen

88. Nail wraps are rebalanced with resin and new fabric after _____ weeks.

   a) Two

   b) Three

   c) Four

   d) Five

89. Nail _____ removes surface moisture and tiny amounts of oil left on the natural nail.

   a) Primer

   b) Dehydrator

   c) Adhesive

   d) Abrasive

90. When you have _____ , you are committed to a strong code of moral and artistic value.

    a) Motivation

    b) Integrity

    c) Work ethic

    d) Enthusiasm

91. A chain of five or more salons owned by one individual or two or more partners is called a/an _____ .

    a) Small independent salon

    b) Independent chain salon

    c) Large national salon chain

    d) Franchise salon

92. When you interview for a job be sure and _____ .

    a) Be late

    b) Project a warm smile

    c) Smoke and/or chew gum

    d) Lean on the interviewer's desk

93. What type of insurance should you purchase when opening your own business?

    _____

    a) Life

    b) Health

    c) Malpractice

    d) Death

94. The very best form of advertising is _____ .

    a) A satisfied client

    b) Radio

    c) Television

    d) Internet

95. _____ is a chemical mixture of concentrated protein and is used to provide treatment when an equal degree of moisturizing and protein is required.

a) Conditioner

b) Deep conditioner

c) Instant conditioner

d) Moisturizing conditioner

96. _____ is rain water or chemically treated water that allows the soap and shampoo to lather freely.

a) Soft water

b) Hard water

c) Acidic water

d) Alkaline water

97. A _____ shampoo contain special chemicals or drugs that are very effective in reducing excessive dandruff.

a) Acid balanced

b) Color-enhancing

c) Medicated

d) Dry/powder

98. _____, usually found in a cream base, are used to soften and improve the health of the scalp.

a) Spray on thermal protectors

b) Scalp conditioners

c) Medicated scalp lotions

d) Scalp astringent lotions

99. A change in the physical properties of a substance without the formation of a new substance is _____.

a) A chemical change

b) A physical change

c) A chemical reaction

d) The result of chemical reaction

100. A rate of nail growth of ⅛ inch per month is average for _____.

    a) Infants

    b) Children

    c) Elderly persons

    d) Normal adult

101. To fill in sparse areas of the eyebrows, use _____.

    a) Mascara

    b) Eye shadow

    c) Eyebrow color

    d) Liquid eyeliner

TEST II: MULTIPLE CHOICE TEST

Directions: Carefully read each statement. Circle the word or phrase that correctly completes the statement.

1. The first culture to cultivate beauty in an extravagant fashion were the _____.

   a) Greeks

   b) Romans

   c) English

   d) Egyptians

2. As long ago as 3000 BC, nail care was practiced in _____.

   a) Europe and America

   b) Asia and India

   c) Egypt and China

   d) China and Europe

3. When designing a time management system, make sure it will work for _____.

   a) Yourself

   b) Instructor

   c) Family

   d) Friends

4. A person's physical posture, walk and movements is known as _____.

   a) Ergonomics

   b) Personal hygiene

   c) Physical presentation

   d) Professional image

5. Listening to a client and then repeating, in your own words, what you think the client said is _____.

   a) Clarification

   b) Communication

   c) Client consultation

   d) Reflective listening

6. An agency that exists to protect the consumers' health, safety, and welfare while receiving services in the salon is the _____.

   a) MSDS

   b) OSHA

   c) State Board

   d) EPA

7. _____ are one-celled microorganisms with both plant and animal characteristics.

   a) Bacteria

   b) Fungus

   c) Virus

   d) Toxins

8. A disease that is communicable or easily spread by contact is a/an _____.

   a) Contaminant

   b) Contagious disease

   c) Infection

   d) Allergy

9. A powerful disinfectant that has a very high pH and can cause damage to the skin and eyes is a/an _____.

   a) Phenolics

   b) Alcohol

   c) Household bleach

   d) Fumigant

10. The study of the functions and activities performed by the body structures is
_____.

   a) Anatomy

   b) Physiology

   c) Histology

   d) Biology

11. A chemical process that takes place in living organisms where cells are nourished and carry out their activities is _____.

   a) Cell membrane

   b) Cytoplasm

   c) Metabolism

   d) Anabolism

12. The hindmost bone of the skull is the _____.

   a) Parietal bone

   b) Occipital bone

   c) Frontal bone

   d) Temporal bone

13. The large, flat, triangular bone of the shoulder is the _____ bone.

   a) Thorax

   b) Scapula

   c) Hyoid

   d) Sternum

14. The bones in the palm of the hand are the _____.

   a) Metacarpus

   b) Carpus

   c) Phalanges

   d) Radius

15. The muscle of the neck that lowers and rotates the head is the _____.

 a) Auricularis posterious

 b) Auricularis anterior

 c) Sternocleidomastoideus

 d) Orbicularis oculi

16. The _____ nerve with its branches affects the little finger side of the arm and palm of the hand.

 a) Median

 b) Ulnar

 c) Radial

 d) Digital

17. The study of the structure, function, and disease of the muscles is _____.

 a) Myology

 b) Biology

 c) Physiology

 d) Neurology

18. The outermost layer of the skin is the _____.

 a) Subcutaneous

 b) Dermis

 c) Adipose

 d) Epidermis

19. A fatty layer found below the dermis is the _____.

 a) Subcutaneous tissue

 b) Dermis

 c) Epidermis

 d) True skin

20. The best source for vitamin _____ is the sunlight.

    a) A

    b) B

    c) C

    d) D

21. Drinking pure water sustains the health of the cells, aids in the elimination of toxins and waste, helps regulate body temperature, and aids in proper _____.

    a) Metabolism

    b) Congestion

    c) Digestion

    d) Respiration

22. The nail is an appendage of the skin and is part of the _____.

    a) Integumentary system

    b) Skeletal system

    c) Muscular system

    d) Nervous system

23. _____ is a touch bank of fibrous tissue that connects bones or holds an organ in place.

    a) Hyponychium

    b) Ligament

    c) Matrix

    d) Cuticle

24. Portion of the skin that supports the nail plate as it grows toward the free edge.

    _____

    a) Nail groove

    b) Nail fold

    c) Nail plate

    d) Nail bed

25. The lowest area or part of the hair strand is the _____ .

    a) Hair bulb

    b) Dermal papilla

    c) Follicle

    d) Hair shaft

26. A weak physical side bond that is easily broken by water or heat is a _____ bond.

    a) Cysteine

    b) Side

    c) Disulfide

    d) Hydrogen

27. Hair loss that is characterized by the sudden falling out of hair in round patches or baldness in spots is _____ .

    a) Postpartum alopecia

    b) Alopecia areata

    c) Alopecia

    d) Androgenic alopecia

28. A type of fungal infection characterized by red papules or spots at the opening of the hair follicles is _____ .

    a) Tinea favosa

    b) Tinea capitis

    c) Scabies

    d) Pediculosis capitis

29. _____ is the technical term for brittle hair.

    a) Hypertrichosis

    b) Trichoptilosis

    c) Trichorrhexis nodosa

    d) Fragilitas crinium

30. A _____ is an unstable mixture of undissolved particles in a liquid.

   a) Solute

   b) Solution

   c) Solvent

   d) Suspension

31. _____ has a pH below 7 and contract and harden the hair.

   a) Acid

   b) Alkalis

   c) Oxidizer

   d) Base

32. The rapid oxidation of substance, accompanied by the production of heat and light is

   _____ .

   a) Oxidation

   b) Combustion

   c) Exothermic

   d) Endothermic

33. A substance that does not easily transmit electricity is a/an _____ .

   a) Current

   b) Conductor

   c) Insulator

   d) Circuit

34. An applicator for directing the electric current from the machine to the client's skin is
   a/an _____ .

   a) Cathode

   b) Polarity

   c) Electrode

   d) Anode

35. The process of introducing water-soluble products into the skin with the use of electric current is _____.

 a) Cataphoresis

 b) Anaphoresis

 c) Iontophoresis

 d) Disincrustation

36. The outline or silhouette of a hairstyle is known as the _____.

 a) Line

 b) Design

 c) Form

 d) Space

37. Lines positioned between horizontal and vertical are _____.

 a) Vertical

 b) Horizontal

 c) Diagonal

 d) Curved

38. Lighter and warmer colors are used to create the illusion of _____.

 a) Repetition

 b) Closeness

 c) Volume

 d) Width

39. The pattern that creates movement in a hairstyle is known as _____.

 a) Balance

 b) Rhythm

 c) Harmony

 d) Emphasis

40. The profile which has a receding forehead and chin is called the _____ profile.

    a) Convex

    b) Concave

    c) Curved

    d) Straight

41. A system for understanding the relationships of color is called _____.

    a) The Law of Color

    b) The level system

    c) The color wheel

    d) Primary color system

42. An example of a natural or vegetable haircolor obtained from the leaves or bark of plants is _____.

    a) Tint

    b) Toner

    c) Metallic

    d) Henna

43. Colors achieved by mixing equal parts of two primary colors are called _____.

    a) Secondary

    b) Tertiary

    c) Complementary

    d) Neutral

44. The melanin found in red hair is known as _____.

    a) Pheomelanin

    b) Eumelanin

    c) Euromelanin

    d) Neomelanin

45. The measure of the potential oxidation of varying strengths of hydrogen peroxide is

_____ .

a) Density

b) Value

c) Volume

d) Percentage

46. The process of treating gray or very resistant hair to allow for better penetration of color is known as _____ .

a) Presoftening

b) Prelightening

c) Activating

d) Accelerating

47. What are the three types of lighteners? _____

a) Cream, paste, powder

b) Cream, paste, oil

c) Oil, cream, powder

d) Oil, paste, powder

48. An abnormal rounded, solid lump above, within or under the skin that is larger than a papule is a _____ .

a) Tubercle

b) Wheal

c) Bulla

d) Macule

49. A skin disease characterized by red patches, covered with silver white scales is

_____ .

a) Dermatitis

b) Exzema

c) Psoriasis

d) Herpes simplex

50. Foul-smelling perspiration is called _____.

    a) Anhidrosis

    b) Bromhidrosis

    c) Hypertrichosis

    d) Chloasma

51. A healthy nail appears slightly _____ in color.

    a) Yellow

    b) Pink

    c) Blue

    d) Purple

52. The lifting of the nail plate from the nail bed, without shedding, is _____.

    a) Onychophagy

    b) Onychorrhexis

    c) Onycholysis

    d) Onychocryptosis

53. The medical term for fungal infections of the feet is _____.

    a) Plicatured nail

    b) Pyogenic granuloma

    c) Pincer nail

    d) Tinea pedis

54. Visible depressions running across the width of the natural nail plate are _____.

    a) Ridges

    b) Leukonychia

    c) Melanonychia

    d) Beau's lines

55. The area between the apex and back of the parietal ridge is the _____.

   a) Crown

   b) Nape

   c) Bang

   d) Crest

56. A styling or cutting comb is called a/an _____ comb.

   a) All purpose

   b) Barber

   c) Tint

   d) Wide-tooth

57. A _____ is a graduated effect achieved by cutting the hair with elevation or overdirection.

   a) Blunt cut

   b) Graduate cut

   c) Layered cut

   d) Long layered cut

58. A technique that removes bulk and adds movement through the lengths of the hair is _____.

   a) Carving

   b) Slicing

   c) Notching

   d) Point cutting

59. The stationary foundation of a pin curl is the closest to the scalp _____.

   a) Base

   b) Stem

   c) Circle

   d) Curl

60. _____ base pin curls are recommended along the front or facial hairline to prevent breaks or splits in the finished hairstyle.

    a) Rectangular

    b) Triangular

    c) Arc

    d) Square

61. For the least volume, the _____ roller sits completely off the base.

    a) On base

    b) Half base

    c) Full base

    d) Off base

62. _____ brushes are well suited for mid to longer length hair.

    a) Paddle

    b) Vent

    c) Round

    d) Grooming

63. _____ irons have straight edges used to create smooth, straight styles.

    a) Curling

    b) Flat

    c) Thermal

    d) Electrical

64. _____ provide a strong curl with full volume.

    a) Full base curls

    b) Half base curls

    c) Off base curls

    d) Finished curls

65. A _____ braid is a three-strand braid that employs the underhand technique.

   a) Invisible

   b) Visible

   c) Fish tail

   d) Rope

66. _____ wigs are constructed with an elasticized mesh fiber base to which the hair is attached.

   a) Cap

   b) Capless

   c) Wefts

   d) Hand-tied

67. A simple quick stitch used to secure the entire length of the weft to the track is

   _____.

   a) Lock stitch

   b) Double lock stitch

   c) Overcast stitch

   d) Single stitch

68. _____ uses intense light to destroy the growth cells of the hair follicles.

   a) Photo-epilation

   b) Electrolysis

   c) Laser

   d) Sugaring

69. A temporary hair removal method that is practiced in many Eastern cultures _____.

   a) Shaving

   b) Waxing

   c) Tweezing

   d) Threading

70. _____ hair is the most common hair texture and does not pose any special problems in chemical hair texture services.

    a) Coarse

    b) Medium

    c) Fine

    d) Thick

71. The _____ end wrap uses one end paper folded in half over the hair ends like an envelope.

    a) Double flat wrap

    b) Single flat wrap

    c) Bookend wrap

    d) Base section wrap

72. _____ is a chemical reaction that heats up the solution and speeds up processing.

    a) Endothermic

    b) Exothermic

    c) Acid-balanced

    d) Alkaline

73. _____ permanently rearranges the structure of curly hair into a straighter or smoother form.

    a) Thermal pressing

    b) Thermal waving

    c) Chemical hair relaxing

    d) Permanent waving

74. An _____ chemical reaction is one that absorbs heat from an outside source.

    a) Endothermic

    b) Exothermic

    c) Acid-balanced

    d) Alkaline

75. _____ is a skin condition where dark blotches of color are most often caused by the sun or hormone imbalances.

    a) Hyperpigmentation

    b) Dehydration

    c) Rosacea

    d) Sun-damaged

76. Masks most often used for oily and combination skin are _____.

    a) Clay masks

    b) Gel masks

    c) Alginate masks

    d) Paraffin masks

77. _____ consists of short, quick tapping, slapping, and hacking movements.

    a) Petrissage

    b) Effleurage

    c) Friction

    d) Tapotement

78. A cosmetic used to outline and emphasize the eyes is _____.

    a) Mascara

    b) Eyeliner

    c) Eyebrow pencils

    d) Eye shadow

79. A jaw that is wider than the forehead characterizes the _____ face.

    a) Round

    b) Square

    c) Triangular

    d) Inverted triangle

80. _____ eyes can be made to appear closer together by extending the eyebrow line to the inside corners of the eyes.

   a) Round

   b) Close set

   c) Wide set

   d) Heavy lidded

81. The _____ pusher is used to push back the eponychium and to gently scrape cuticle tissue from the natural nail plate.

   a) Metal pusher

   b) Metal file

   c) Wooden pusher

   d) Orangewood stick

82. The _____ creates a colorless layer on the natural nail that improves adhesion of polish.

   a) Top coat

   b) Base coat

   c) Nail hardener

   d) Nail conditioner

83. The _____ has a free edge that is rounded off and should extend only slightly past the finger tip.

   a) Square nail

   b) Squoval nail

   c) Round nail

   d) Pointed nail

84. The _____ is very stimulating and increases blood flow.

   a) Friction movement

   b) Effleurage

   c) Kneading movement

   d) Wringing

85. A product(s) containing gentle soaps and moisturizers that are used in a pedicure bath to clean and soften the skin is/are _____ .

    a) Abrasive scrubs

    b) Callus softeners

    c) Paraffin wax

    d) Foot soaks

86. An _____ has a rough surface used to shape or smooth the nail and remove surface shine.

    a) Abrasive board

    b) Emery board

    c) Buffer block

    d) Three-way buffer

87. A thick, natural material with a tight weave that becomes transparent when resin is applied is _____ .

    a) Silk

    b) Fiberglas

    c) Fabric

    d) Linen

88. Additives designed to speed up chemical reactions are _____ .

    a) Monomers

    b) Polymers

    c) Initiators

    d) Catalysts

89. Nail _____ is used for securing nail tips to the natural nails.

    a) Primer

    b) Dehydrator

    c) Adhesive

    d) Abrasive

90. _____ is eagerness to learn, grow, and expand your skills and knowledge.

    a) Motivation

    b) Integrity

    c) Work ethic

    d) Enthusiasm

91. A/n _____ is often located in busy, low-rent shopping center strips that are anchored by a nearby supermarket or other large business.

    a) Basic value priced salon

    b) Mid priced full service salon

    c) High-end salon

    d) Image or day spa

92. A question that an interviewer can not ask you by law is _____.

    a) Are you able to perform the job?

    b) In which languages are you fluent?

    c) How old are you?

    d) Are you authorized to work in the United States?

93. A _____ is two or more people sharing ownership.

    a) Individual

    b) Partnership

    c) Corporation

    d) Stockholders

94. A shampoo that washes away excess oiliness from oily hair and scalp, while keeping the hair from drying out is a/an _____.

    a) Acid-balanced shampoo

    b) Balancing shampoo

    c) Clarifying shampoo

    d) Color-enhancing shampoo

95. _____ is a special chemical agent applied to the hair to deposit protein or moisture, help restore its strength, and give it body.

   a) Conditioner

   b) Deep conditioner

   c) Instant conditioner

   d) Moisturizing conditioner

96. The end of the surfactant molecule that is a water-attracting head is a _____.

   a) Detergent

   b) Surfactant

   c) Hydrophilic

   d) Lipophilic

97. A _____ shampoo is used to brighten and add a slight hint of color to the hair and to eliminate unwanted color tones such as gold or brassiness.

   a) Acid balanced

   b) Color-enhancing

   c) Medicated

   d) Dry/powder

98. Pathogenic bacteria are _____.

   a) Harmless

   b) Unimportant

   c) Helpful

   d) Harmful

99. The lightness or darkness of color is measured in terms of _____.

   a) Level

   b) Tone

   c) Intensity

   d) Contributing pigment

100. Cleansing the hair and scalp is the primary purpose of _____.

    a) Shampooing in the salon

    b) An appointment at the salon

    c) The use of conditioner

    d) A day at the spa

TEST III: MULTIPLE CHOICE TEST

Directions: Carefully read each statement. Circle the word or phrase that correctly completes the statement.

1. In ancient Rome, a woman's status was indicated by _____ .

   a) Haircolor

   b) Nail color

   c) Eye color

   d) Makeup

2. By developing a game plan you are _____ .

   a) Wasting your time

   b) Consciously planning your life

   c) Procrastinating

   d) Being selfish

3. Clean, fresh smelling and well maintained clothes are a part of _____ .

   a) Ethics

   b) Good personal hygiene

   c) Good personal grooming

   d) Positive attitude

4. The study of how a workplace can best be designed for comfort, safety, efficiency and productivity is _____ .

   a) Ergonomics

   b) Professionalism

   c) Physical presentation

   d) Professional image

5. The act of accurately sharing information between two people or groups of people is called _____.

   a) Clarification

   b) Communication

   c) Client consultation

   d) Reflective Listening

6. An organism that lives on or in another organism and draws its nourishment from that organism is a _____.

   a) Bacteria

   b) Virus

   c) Toxin

   d) Parasite

7. An immune system response to certain foods, chemicals, product ingredients or other normally harmless substances is a/an _____.

   a) Contaminant

   b) Contagious disease

   c) Infection

   d) Allergy

8. Sodium hypochlorite is commonly known as _____.

   a) Phenolics

   b) Alcohol

   c) Household bleach

   d) Fumigant

9. The basic unit of all living things is _____.

   a) Nerves

   b) Cells

   c) Tissues

   d) Nucleus

10. _____ tissue, such as blood and lymph, carries food, waste products, and hormones through the body.

   a) Connective

   b) Epithelial

   c) Liquid

   d) Muscular

11. The _____ bone forms the forehead.

   a) Parietal

   b) Occipital

   c) Frontal

   d) Temporal

12. The small, thin bones located at the front inner wall of the orbits is the _____ bone.

   a) Lacrimal

   b) Nasal

   c) Maxillae

   d) Mandible

13. Muscles that are involuntary and function automatically, without conscious will are the _____ muscles.

   a) Striated

   b) Nonstriated

   c) Cardiac

   d) Skeletal

14. The large, triangular muscle covering the shoulder joint that allows the arm to extend outward and to the side of the body is the _____ .

   a) Bicep

   b) Deltoid

   c) Tricep

   d) Flexors

15. The tiny, thin-walled blood vessels that connect the smaller arteries to the veins are

_____ .

   a) Capillaries

   b) Arteries

   c) Veins

   d) Vessels

16. The ring muscle of the eye socket, enabling you to close your eyes is the _____ .

   a) Auricularis posterious

   b) Auricularis anterior

   c) Sternocleidomastoideus

   d) Orbicularis oculi

17. Which layer of the skin contains numerous blood vessels, lymph vessels, nerves, sweat and oil glands, and hair follicles? _____

   a) Subcutaneous

   b) Dermis

   c) Adipose

   d) Epidermis

18. No oil glands are found here. _____

   a) Forehead

   b) Face

   c) Scalp

   d) Palms

19. The secretory nerves are part of the _____ system.

   a) Respiratory

   b) Autonomic nervous

   c) Circulatory

   d) Excretory

20. Small epidermal structures with nerve endings that are sensitive to touch and pressure are _____.

   a) Sudoriferous glands

   b) Sebaceous glands

   c) Subcutaneous tissue

   d) Tactile corpuscles

21. Thickened skin between the fingertip and free edge of the nail plate is the _____.

   a) Hyponychium

   b) Eponyichium

   c) Bed epithelium

   d) Nail grooves

22. The portion of the skin that supports the nail plate as it grows toward the free edge is the _____.

   a) Nail groove

   b) Nail fold

   c) Nail plate

   d) Nail unit

23. The tube like depression or pocket in the skin or scalp that contains the hair root is the _____.

   a) Hair bulb

   b) Dermal papilla

   c) Follicle

   d) Hair shaft

24. The middle layer of the hair is the _____.

   a) Cuticle

   b) Cortex

   c) Medulla

   d) Keratin

25. Hair _____ is the thickness or diameter of the individual hair strand.

   a) Diameter

   b) Porosity

   c) Texture

   d) Elasticity

26. The technical term for gray hair is _____.

   a) Hypertrichosis

   b) Monilethrix

   c) Canities

   d) Pityriasis

27. The infestation of the hair and scalp with head lice is _____.

   a) Tinea favosa

   b) Tinea capitis

   c) Scabies

   d) Pediculosis capitis

28. Anything that occupies space and has mass is _____.

   a) Matter

   b) Atoms

   c) Elements

   d) Molecules

29. A/an _____ is an unstable mixture of two or more immiscible substances united with the aid of an emulsifier.

   a) Emulsion

   b) Surfactant

   c) Hydrophilic

   d) Lipophilic

30. _____ has a pH above 7 and softens and swells the hair and skin.

    a) Acid

    b) Alkalis

    c) Oxidizer

    d) Base

31. The chemical reaction that combines a substance with oxygen to produce an oxide is _____ .

    a) Oxidation

    b) Combustion

    c) Exothermic

    d) Endothermic

32. A unit that measures the pressure of force that pushes the flow of electrons forward through a conductor is a/an _____.

    a) Volt

    b) Amp

    c) Ohm

    d) Watt

33. A _____ current is a constant and direct current having a positive and negative pole, producing chemical changes when it passes through the tissues and fluids of the body.

    a) Galvanic

    b) Faradic

    c) Sinusoidal

    d) Tesla-high frequency

34. _____ is the process used to soften and emulsify grease deposits and blackheads in the hair follicles.

    a) Cataphoresis

    b) Anaphoresis

    c) Iontophoresis

    d) Disincrustation

35. The area the hairstyle occupies is called _____.

    a) Line

    b) Design

    c) Form

    d) Space

36. An example of a line that is found in the one-length hairstyle is the _____.

    a) Single line

    b) Transitional line

    c) Contrasting line

    d) Repeating line

37. Curly hair can be permanently straightened with _____.

    a) Hair relaxers

    b) Curling irons

    c) Flat irons

    d) Pressing irons

38. The _____ in a hairstyle is the place the eyes see first.

    a) Balance

    b) Rhythm

    c) Harmony

    d) Emphasis

39. The profile which has a prominent forehead and chin is the _____ profile.

    a) Convex

    b) Concave

    c) Curved

    d) Straight

40. A mixture of shampoo, permanent haircolor, and hydrogen peroxide creates a

    _____ .

    a) Soap cap

    b) Highlighting shampoo

    c) Color filler

    d) Highlighting shampoo tint

41. Colored mousse and gels are considered to be what haircolor category?_____

    a) Temporary

    b) Semipermanent

    c) Demipermanent

    d) Permanent

42. Primary and secondary colors that are positioned opposite each other on the color wheel
    are considered to be _____ .

    a) Secondary

    b) Tertiary

    c) Complementary

    d) Neutral

43. The melanin that gives black and brown color to hair is known as _____ .

    a) Pheomelanin

    b) Eumelanin

    c) Euromelanin

    d) Neomelanin

44. The preliminary strand test will tell you how the hair will react to the color formula and
    indicate _____ .

    a) Processing time

    b) Application method

    c) Client satisfaction

    d) Application time

45. What is added to hydrogen peroxide to increase its chemical action or lifting power?

_____

   a) Accelerator

   b) Diffuser

   c) Dissolver

   d) Activator

46. Which type of lightener is not used directly on the scalp? _____

   a) Cream

   b) Paste

   c) Oil

   d) Powder

47. A condition of dry, scaly skin characterized by absolute or partial deficiency of sebum is _____ .

   a) Asteatosis

   b) Seborrhea

   c) Steatoma

   d) Rosacea

48. A term used to indicate an inflammatory condition of the skin is _____ .

   a) Dermatitis

   b) Eczema

   c) Psoriasis

   d) Herpes simplex

49. Deficiency in perspiration is called _____ .

   a) Anhidrosis

   b) Bromhidrosis

   c) Hypertrichosis

   d) Chloasma

50. An inflammation of the matrix of the nail with a shedding of the nail is _____

    a) Onychocryptosis

    b) Onychia

    c) Onychophagy

    d) Onychomycosis

51. The technical term for bitten nails is _____ .

    a) Onychophagy

    b) Onychorrhexis

    c) Onycholysis

    d) Onychocryptosis

52. A condition in which a blood clot forms under the nail plate, forming a dark purplish spot, usually due to injury _____ .

    a) Eggshell nail

    b) Bruised nail

    c) Melanonychia

    d) Nail pterygium

53. The _____ is the widest area on the head, starting at the temples and ending at the bottom of the crown.

    a) Occipital

    b) Apex

    c) Parietal ridge

    d) Four corners

54. The _____ is the angle at which the fingers are held when cutting, the line that is cut creating the end shape.

    a) Guideline

    b) Perimeters

    c) Cutting line

    d) Subsection

55. When cutting with a vertical or diagonal cutting line, cutting _____ is the best way to maintain control of the subsection.

   a) Over your fingers

   b) Below the fingers

   c) Palm to palm

   d) Palm to knuckles

56. _____ is a technique performed on the ends of the hair using the tips or points of the shears.

   a) Notching

   b) Free-hand notching

   c) Slithering

   d) Point cutting

57. A version of slicing that creates a visual separation in the hair is _____.

   a) Carving

   b) Slicing

   c) Notching

   d) Point cutting

58. The section of the pin curl, that gives the curl its direction and movement _____.

   a) Base

   b) Stem

   c) Circle

   d) Curl

59. _____ base pin curls are suitable for curly hairstyles without much volume or lift.

   a) Rectangular

   b) Triangular

   c) Arc

   d) Square

60. _____ is used to keep curly hair smooth and straight, while still retaining a beautiful shape.

   a) Hair wrapping

   b) Blow drying

   c) Velcro rollers

   d) Flat iron

61. A thick styling preparation that comes in a tube or bottle is _____ .

   a) Gel

   b) Mousse

   c) Pomade

   d) Volumizer

62. _____ provide maximum lift or volume.

   a) End curls

   b) Volume thermal curls

   c) Volume base curls

   d) Full base curls

63. _____ is a manufactured synthetic fiber or excellent quality for braiding.

   a) Nylon

   b) Rayon

   c) Lin

   d) Kanekalon

64. The _____ braid is made with two strands that are twisted around each other.

   a) Invisible

   b) Visible

   c) Fish tail

   d) Rope

65. _____ wigs are machine made.

   a) Cap

   b) Capless

   c) Wefts

   d) Hand-tied

66. In the _____ method of attaching extensions, the extension is bonded to the client's own hair with a bonding material that is activated by the heat from a special tool.

   a) Glue

   b) Adhesive

   c) Bonding

   d) Fusion

67. The most common form of temporary hair removal is _____.

   a) Shaving

   b) Waxing

   c) Tweezing

   d) Threading

68. The _____ is the innermost layer of the hair and is often called the pith or core of the hair.

   a) Cortex

   b) Medulla

   c) Cuticle

   d) Shaft

69. When analyzing the hair for a chemical hair service, the _____ of the hair determines its ability to hold a curl and is more important than any other single factor.

   a) Texture

   b) Density

   c) Porosity

   d) Elasticity

70. The method of wrapping a permanent wave from the ends to the scalp is a _____ wrap.

   a) Spiral

   b) Directional

   c) Bricklay

   d) Croquignole

71. The perm wrap where base sections are offset from each other row by row, to prevent noticeable splits and blend the flow of the hair is a _____.

   a) Basic perm wrap

   b) Curvature perm wrap

   c) Bricklay wrap

   d) Spiral wrap

72. The oldest and most common type of chemical hair relaxers is _____.

   a) Metal hydroxide

   b) Sodium hydroxide

   c) Guanidine relaxer

   d) Lithium hydroxide

73. Skin with very small pores that may be dehydrated with fine lines and wrinkles and is dry and rough to the touch is _____.

   a) Oily skin

   b) Dry skin

   c) Combination

   d) Acne

74. _____ is a chronic hereditary disorder that can be indicated by constant or frequent facial blushing.

   a) Hyperpigmentation

   b) Dehydration

   c) Rosacea

   d) Sun-damaged

75. _____ are often seaweed based.

    a) Clay masks

    b) Gel masks

    c) Alginate masks

    d) Paraffin masks

76. _____, a type of mechanical exfoliation, uses a closed vacuum to shoot crystals onto the skin, bumping off cell buildup that is then vacuumed by the suction.

    a) Galvanic

    b) High frequency

    c) Electrotherapy

    d) Microdermabrasion

77. A _____ brush is a large, soft brush used for blending the edges of color.

    a) Blush

    b) Concealer

    c) Eye shadow

    d) Powder

78. The _____ face has a wide forehead and narrow, pointed chin.

    a) Round

    b) Square

    c) Triangular

    d) Inverted triangle

79. Eyelash hairs on a strip that are applied with adhesive to the natural lash line are called _____ .

    a) Individual lashes

    b) Band lashes

    c) Eye tabbing

    d) Group lashes

80. A _____ is used to clean fingernails and to remove dust and debris with warm soapy water.

   a) Tweezers

   b) Cuticle scissors

   c) Cuticle nippers

   d) Nail brush

81. _____ are used to improve the durability of weak or thin nail plates.

   a) Top coat

   b) Base coat

   c) Nail hardener

   d) Nail conditioner

82. The _____ should be slightly tapered and extended just a bit past the tip of the finger.

   a) Square nail

   b) Squoval nail

   c) Round nail

   d) Pointed nail

83. A _____ is a metal file designed to file in one direction.

   a) Nail file

   b) Nail rasp

   c) Foot file

   d) Nippers

84. An instrument used for manicures and pedicures to trim tags of dead skin is a

   _____ .

   a) Nail file

   b) Nail rasp

   c) Foot file

   d) Nippers

85. A lightweight rectangular block used to buff nails is a _____ .

   a) Abrasive board

   b) Emery board

   c) Buffer block

   d) Three-way buffer

86. Nail wraps must be rebalanced with additional resin after _____ weeks.

   a) Two

   b) Three

   c) Four

   d) Five

87. An _____ starts a chain reaction that leads to the creation of long polymer chains.

   a) Monomer

   b) Polymer

   c) Initiator

   d) Catalyst

88. Ultraviolet gel enhancements must be rebalanced every _____ weeks.

   a) 1 to 2

   b) 2 to 3

   c) 3 to 4

   d) 4 to 5

89. _____ means having the drive to take the necessary action to achieve a goal.

   a) Motivation

   b) Integrity

   c) Work ethic

   d) Enthusiasm

90. When writing a resume, you should _____ .

    a) Stretch the truth

    b) Include personal references

    c) Reference salaries

    d) Keep it short

91. A _____ is a percentage of the revenue that the salon takes in and is usually offered to practitioners once they have built up a loyal clientele.

    a) Salary

    b) Hourly

    c) Commission

    d) Salary plus commission

92. The nerve center of the salon is in the _____ .

    a) Break room

    b) Shampoo area

    c) Reception area

    d) Dispensary

93. A shampoo that contains an acidic ingredient to cut through product buildup that can flatten hair is a/an _____ .

    a) Acid-balanced shampoo

    b) Balancing shampoo

    c) Clarifying shampoo

    d) Color-enhancing shampoo

94. _____ is often in well water and contains certain minerals that lessen the ability of soap or shampoo to lather readily.

    a) Soft water

    b) Hard water

    c) Acidic water

    d) Alkaline water

95. The end of the surfactant molecule that is an oil attracting tail is a _____ .

   a) Detergent

   b) Surfactant

   c) Hydrophilic

   d) Lipophilic

96. _____ remove oil accumulation from the scalp and are used after a scalp treatment, before styling.

   a) Spray on thermal protectors

   b) Scalp conditioners

   c) Medicated scalp lotions

   d) Scalp astringent lotions

97. Chemicals can be used to alter _____ .

   a) Face shape

   b) Skin tone

   c) Wave patterns

   d) Hair density

98. Bleaching or decolorizing is also called _____ .

   a) Uncoloring

   b) Lightening

   c) Lowlightening

   d) Stripping

99. The primary colors are red, yellow, and _____ .

   a) Black

   b) Green

   c) Orange

   d) Blue

100. To fill in sparse areas of the eyebrows, use _____ .

    a) Mascara

    b) Eye shadow

    c) Eyebrow color

    d) Liquid eyeliner

ANATOMY TEST: MULTIPLE CHOICE TEST

Directions: Carefully read each statement. Circle the word or phrase that correctly completes the statement.

1. The study of the structure of the human body that can be seen with the naked eye is
   _____.

   a) Anatomy

   b) Physiology

   c) Histology

   d) Biology

2. _____ is the study of tiny structures found in living tissue that is
   microscopic anatomy.

   a) Anatomy

   b) Physiology

   c) Histology

   d) Biology

3. The dense, active protoplasm found in the center of the cell is the _____.

   a) Nerves

   b) Cells

   c) Tissues

   d) Nucleus

4. The _____ is all the protoplasm of a cell that surrounds the nucleus.

   a) Cell membrane

   b) Cytoplasm

   c) Metabolism

   d) Anabolism

5. A collection of similar cells that perform a particular function is _____ .

   a) Organs

   b) Cells

   c) Tissues

   d) Muscles

6. _____ tissue serves to support, protect, and bind together other tissues of the body.

   a) Connective

   b) Epithelial

   c) Liquid

   d) Muscular

7. _____ tissue are a protective covering on the body surfaces.

   a) Connective

   b) Epithelial

   c) Liquid

   d) Muscular

8. _____ tissue contracts and moves the various parts of the body.

   a) Connective

   b) Epithelial

   c) Liquid

   d) Muscular

9. Groups of tissues designed to perform a specific function are _____ .

   a) Organs

   b) Cells

   c) Tissues

   d) Muscles

10. The cranium is made up of _____ bones.

    a) Two

    b) Four

    c) Six

    d) Eight

11. The two _____ bones form the sides and crown of the cranium.

    a) Parietal

    b) Occipital

    c) Frontal

    d) Temporal

12. The main bone of the neck is the _____ bone and the cervical vertebrae.

    a) Thorax

    b) Scapula

    c) Hyoid

    d) Sternum

13. The _____ is the bony cage that serves as a protective framework for the heart, lungs, and other internal organs.

    a) Thorax

    b) Scapula

    c) Hyoid

    d) Sternum

14. The breastbone, the flat bone that forms the ventral support of the ribs, is the _____ bone.

    a) Thorax

    b) Scapula

    c) Hyoid

    d) Sternum

15. The two _____ bones form the bridge of the nose.

   a) Lacrimal

   b) Nasal

   c) Maxillae

   d) Mandible

16. The _____ is the lower jawbone and is the largest and strongest bone of the face.

   a) Lacrimal

   b) Nasal

   c) Maxillae

   d) Mandible

17. The two _____ bones form the upper jaw.

   a) Lacrimal

   b) Nasal

   c) Maxillae

   d) Mandible

18. The inner and larger bone of the forearm is the _____ .

   a) Ulna

   b) Radius

   c) Carpus

   d) Humerus

19. Bones in the fingers are the _____ .

   a) Metacarpus

   b) Carpus

   c) Phalanges

   d) Radius

20. The body system that covers, shapes, and supports the skeleton tissue is the
_____ system.

   a) Muscular

   b) Skeletal

   c) Circulatory

   d) Nervous

21. Muscles that are attached to the bones and are voluntary are the _____
muscles.

   a) Striated

   b) Nonstriated

   c) Cardiac

   d) Smooth

22. This type of muscle is involuntary and is the only one found in the body _____ .

   a) Striated

   b) Nonstriated

   c) Cardiac

   d) Skeletal

23. The broad muscle that covers the top of the skull is the _____ .

   a) Aponeurosis

   b) Epicranius

   c) Masseter

   d) Platysma

24. The _____ and the temporalis are the muscles that coordinate the
opening and closing of the mouth.

   a) Aponeurosis

   b) Epicranius

   c) Masseter

   d) Platysma

25. The _____ is the broad muscle extending from the chest and shoulder muscles to the side of the chin.

   a) Aponeurosis

   b) Epicranius

   c) Masseter

   d) Platysma

26. The muscle in front of the ear that draws the ear forward is the _____.

   a) Auricularis posterious

   b) Auricularis anterior

   c) Sternocleidomastoideus

   d) Orbicularis oculi

27. The ring muscle of the eye socket, enabling you to close your eyes, is the _____ .

   a) Auricularis posterious

   b) Auricularis anterior

   c) Sternocleidomastoideus

   d) Orbicularis oculi

28. The muscle of the chest that assists the swinging movements of the arm is the _____ .

   a) Trapezius

   b) Pectoralis major

   c) Latissimus dorsi

   d) Serratus anterior

29. The _____ muscle covers the back of the neck and upper and middle region of the back.

   a) Trapezius

   b) Pectoralis major

   c) Latissimus dorsi

   d) Serratus anterior

30. The large muscle that covers the entire back of the upper arm and extends to the forearm is the _____ .

    a) Bicep

    b) Deltoid

    c) Triceps

    d) Flexors

31. The _____ system is an exceptionally well-organized system that is responsible for coordinating all of the many activities that are performed both inside and outside of the body.

    a) Muscular

    b) Skeletal

    c) Circulatory

    d) Nervous

32. The scientific study of the structure, function, and pathology of the nervous system is known as _____ .

    a) Myology

    b) Biology

    c) Physiology

    d) Neurology

33. The study of the structure, function, and disease of the muscles is _____ .

    a) Myology

    b) Biology

    c) Physiology

    d) Neurology

34. _____ nerves carry impulses or messages from the sense organs to the brain.

    a) Sensory

    b) Motor

    c) Reflex

    d) Dendrites

35. Nerves that carry impulses from the brain to the muscles are _____ nerves.

   a) Sensory

   b) Motor

   c) Reflex

   d) Dendrites

36. A _____ is an automatic nerve reaction to a stimulus that involves the movement of an impulse.

   a) Sensory

   b) Motor

   c) Reflex

   d) Dendrites

37. The _____ nerve affects the skin of the lower eyelid, side of the nose, upper lip, and mouth.

   a) Infratrochlear

   b) Auriculotemporal

   c) Infraorbital

   d) Superorbital

38. The nerve that affects the muscles of the upper part of the cheek is the

   _____.

   a) Zygomatic nerve

   b) Mandibular nerve

   c) Cervical nerve

   d) Cutaneous nerve

39. The _____ originates at the spinal cord, and their branches supply the muscles and scalp at the back of the head and neck.

   a) Zygomatic nerve

   b) Mandibular nerve

   c) Cervical nerve

   d) Cutaneous nerve

40. The _____ nerve, with its branches, supplies the fingers.

    a) Median

    b) Ulnar

    c) Radial

    d) Digital

41. The _____ system is also referred to as the cardiovascular system and controls the steady circulation of the blood flow.

    a) Muscular

    b) Skeletal

    c) Circulatory

    d) Nervous

42. The upper, thin-walled chamber is the right and left _____ .

    a) Ventricle

    b) Atrium

    c) Valves

    d) Vessels

43. The lower, thick-walled chambers are the right and left _____ .

    a) Ventricle

    b) Atrium

    c) Valves

    d) Vessels

44. Thick-walled, muscular, flexible tubes that carry oxygenated blood away from the heart are the _____ .

    a) Capillaries

    b) Arteries

    c) Veins

    d) Vessels

45. _____ are produced in the red bone marrow and contain hemoglobin.

    a) Platelets

    b) Plasma

    c) White blood cells

    d) Red blood cells

46. The fluid part of the blood _____ .

    a) Platelets

    b) Plasma

    c) White blood cells

    d) Red blood cells

47. The _____ system is made up of a group of specialized glands that affect the growth, development, sexual activities, and health of the entire body.

    a) Endocrine

    b) Digestive

    c) Excretory

    d) Respiratory

48. The system that is responsible for purifying the body by eliminating waste matter is the _____ system.

    a) Endocrine

    b) Digestive

    c) Excretory

    d) Respiratory

49. The _____ system enables breathing and consists of the lungs and air passages.

    a) Integumentary

    b) Digestive

    c) Excretory

    d) Respiratory

50. The _____ system is made up of the skin and its various accessory organs.

    a) Integumentary

    b) Digestive

    c) Excretory

    d) Respiratory